Forgotten Children of the AIDS Epidemic

Forgotten Children of the AIDS Epidemic

Edited by
Shelley Geballe,
Janice Gruendel, and
Warren Andiman

Yale University Press

New Haven and London

Published with assistance from
The Stewart B. McKinney Foundation.

Designed by James J. Johnson.
Set in Stemple Garamond types by
Marathon Typography Service, Inc.
Printed in the United States of America by
Vail-Ballou Press, Binghamton, New York.

A catalogue record for this book is available
from the British Library.

The paper in this book meets the guidelines
for permanence and durability of the
Committee on Production Guidelines for
Book Longevity of the Council on Library
Resources.

10 9 8 7 6 5 4 3 2 1

*Library of Congress Cataloging-in-
Publication Data*

Forgotten children of the AIDS epidemic /
Shelley Geballe, Janice Gruendel, and
Warren Andiman, editors.
    p.   cm
    Includes bibliographical references and
index.
    ISBN 0-300-06270-2 (c). — ISBN 0-300-
06271-0 (p)
    1. Children of AIDS patients.   2. AIDS
(Disease)—Patients—Family relationships.
3. Children of AIDS patients—Services
for.   I. Geballe, Shelley.   II. Gruendel,
Janice.   III. Andiman, Warren.
    [DNLM: 1. Acquired Immuno-
deficiency Syndrome—psychology.
2. Child of Impaired Parents—psychology.
3. Child Welfare.   WD 308 F721   1995]
RA644.A25F67   1995
362.7—dc20
DNLM/DLC
for Library of Congress   94-34758
                                          CIP

Contents

**Part Three   Responding to the Needs of Children and
Youth Affected by AIDS**

Part Four   Voices: Children, Parents, and Caregivers

Foreword

The tragedy of HIV/AIDS grows more profound with each passing year. Many people have focused on children with the disease itself, but far less attention has been paid to the range and extent of devastation that blights the lives of entire families. For every child directly *in*fected, many more are deeply *af*fected by loss of parents, siblings, other crucial caregivers, and all the stabilizing factors that may spell the difference between a healthy childhood and disaster.

This remarkable book brings together in an immensely useful way the expertise and insight of a coalition of diverse professionals whose work has brought them into the realm of HIV/AIDS as the epidemic impacts families directly. While they are concerned, of course, about the capacity of social and health-related institutions to care for children with AIDS or HIV, they deal most importantly with the interests of the many uninfected children and youths caught up in the tragedies of parental illness and loss, the insecurity of caregivers, the ravages of social stigma and resulting enforced secrecy, and despair. The succinct, germane discussions range all the way from children's tendency to assume guilt for the ill fate of their loved ones to the legal realities of placement and adoption. In between, there is a wealth of pragmatic and humane discussion of options for assistance and understanding of the children besieged by this awful epidemic-counterpart of war.

For those who care for children affected by AIDS in any way, this is a practical reference and handbook. For those who care about children and childhood, it is a powerfully written reminder that the cost of walking away from HIV and AIDS will be paid most dearly in the currency of future generations of children whose lives have been distorted and scarred by society's failure to respond.

The diversity of authorship creates a wonderful aggregation and coalescence of expertise; and the collective insight of the professionals who have contributed should prove to be a major beacon—as well as a resource—for those who will have to cope with the needs of the many thousands of children who now need or will soon need help living through the tragedy of AIDS as it blights those they need and love.

JUNE OSBORN, M.D.

Preface

This book had its start in the voices of four women, all infected by HIV, who spoke of their hopes and fears as they reflected upon the uncertain futures that their children would face after their deaths. The voices of these women soon were joined by those of other mothers, of fathers and grandparents, foster and adoptive parents, and of the children themselves. They all spoke about the forgotten children of the AIDS pandemic, *their* children, who were not themselves infected and were fated to survive the AIDS-related deaths of their parents, siblings, friends and neighbors, often in silence and secrecy. The power of their voices gave rise to our involvement in the production of a video documentary, *Mommy, Who'll Take Care of Me?*, about the experience of these forgotten children.

Our research for this documentary quickly confirmed that these children are largely invisible to both the academic and service communities. Uninfected by HIV, they were not viewed as patients by the medical community. Often unable to share their family secrets and losses, they were invisible as well to schools, churches, courts, and community organizations. While the lay press has increasingly published articles about "AIDS orphans," the scholarly literature has been virtually devoid of research concerning the experience of the children being affected by HIV disease. Few professionals seemed to be helping to plan for their futures, or even to recognize that they existed. The continuing invisibility of these AIDS-affected children was impressed upon us in a discussion with Rosa DeLauro, the congressional representative (D.-Connecticut) for many who have worked on this volume. Shown portions of this book, she declared, "You know, these kids aren't even on the radar screen."

This book's primary goal is to place these forgotten children of the AIDS epidemic on the "radar screen" of professionals, public policy makers, and community workers by providing, in one volume, a broad and comprehensive overview of the experience of the children who are *affected* by AIDS.

We envision several audiences for this book. It is written for social workers, teachers, school nurses, attorneys and judges, juvenile justice personnel, and other professionals in community organizations who may not yet understand the many ways that HIV disease affects children who are not themselves infected. It also is intended for professionals who have some background in child mental health but who have not yet had significant experience working with children affected by HIV. The book seeks to inform policy makers at the state and national levels who have the capacity to craft legislative and administrative remedies for some of the problems faced by HIV-affected children and the families who care for them. Finally, we hope this book will help family members struggling with HIV disease and others in our communities to better understand the impact of the disease on the "well" children in the family.

We do not intend this book to be *the* definitive work about AIDS-affected children for all time. Given the current dearth of research on these children, no work could responsibly make that claim. Rather, the book provides a multi-disciplinary overview of what we now know about these children and their needs, and an agenda for policy reform and research over the next several years. We hope that this book will *not* be an enduring work. We trust that its policy recommendations will grow obsolete as they become more fully implemented. We hope that our discussion of the harm that society's continued stigmatization of AIDS causes these children will encourage all of us to look more critically at ourselves and at our biases. Most fundamentally, we fervently hope for a change in the course of the AIDS pandemic, so that we will be proved wrong in our projections of the number of children who will endure life-altering losses while surviving AIDS in their families.

Acknowledgments

The debts that one tallies in writing and editing a book are many, and we must acknowledge a large group of friends who have joined this journey on behalf of children.

To the chapter authors, we offer a standing ovation for meeting so graciously our extremely tight deadlines amid the enormously demanding work they all do in providing service to those about whom we write. All understood the urgency of getting the messages of this book before the widest audience with the greatest speed.

Many have read and commented on portions of this manuscript, including Philip Alcabes, Margaret Bacon, Miriam Berkman, Chet Brodnicki, Elizabeth Bradley, Frank Farrow, Sue Garten, Marcia Robinson Lowry, Nancy Moss, Kathy Ruhf, Mark Schlesinger, B. Joyce Simpson, Judith Solomon, P. Clay Stevens, Martha Stone, and Alan Terl. We thank them for their assistance.

Others have worked with us in the conceptual development of this book, and in associated projects, among them Judy Belk, Lisa Berkman, Sharon Blair, Geri Brooks, Christine Cimini, Donald Cohen, Congresswoman Rosa DeLauro, Bob Francis, Rich Furman, Ron Gould, Ruth Harlow, Sally Horwitz, Phyllis Joffe, Sharon Koletsky, Steve Marans, John McCally, Lucie McKinney, Anne Murphy, Jane Perkins, Larry Rifkin, Betsy Ryan, Congressman Christopher Shays, the Rev. William Shiflet, Gary Smith, Mark Sottnick, Deborah Wallace, and Edward Zigler.

For their help in giving voice to the children, we thank Larraine Ahto, Lela Charney, Barbara Colley, Barbara Marks, Roxanne Rae, and Florence Samperi. Pamela Loman assisted greatly with the Resource Guide.

We thank Jean Black, science editor at Yale University Press, for shepherding this project through the Press in record time. We thank the anonymous reviewers for their insightful critique of the manuscript and Dan Heaton for his wonderful help in editing. We also thank the Stewart B. McKinney Foundation for financial assistance in reproducing the children's artwork in this volume.

Our families especially deserve our thanks for their patience in enduring our absences, covering for us on the home front, and providing a shoulder to lean on as the pain of these children became ever so real. Thanks to Gordon, Josh, Ben, and Dan; to Herb, David, Darren and Stephen; and to Marie, Sarah, and Alexis. Thanks, too, to Becky for her unknowing role in inspiring this effort.

The final thanks must go to those who have opened their lives and their hearts to us. They have taught us about this illness, given us lessons in coping and resilience, and shared their stories of living with HIV disease in a country that still largely scorns rather than embraces them. As a testament to their generosity and courage, may this book play some small role in changing all that. Thanks to Michael, Venus, Onivea, Bill, Gary, Patsy, "Matthew," Marva, "Kara," "Ann," "Grace," and to the many patients, family members, and friends who wish to remain anonymous.

Forgotten Children of the AIDS Epidemic

Introduction

Little Jackie Johnson's mom, dying of AIDS, had tried to comfort the child, reassuring her that there is a wonderful place called heaven that people go to when they leave this life. . . . On Tuesday, Jackie told companions she wanted to be an angel so she could greet her mother at heaven's gate—and calmly stepped in front of a freight train. Police said her protesting brother and sister tried hard to pull her out of harm's way, but an insistent Jackie fought them off.

The Daily News, New York, June 17, 1993

In the next six years, AIDS will kill the mothers of enough American children to fill the city of Gainesville.

St. Petersburg *Times*, November 14, 1993

A 10-year-old boy fatally shot a classmate because he was persistently teased about his mother having AIDS, the Montana Standard reported Thursday. The shooting killed an 11-year-old boy standing next to the intended victim. The boy's mother . . . lies in a Montana hospital bed dying of acquired immune deficiency syndrome. The boy's father, who has had custody of the child, has the virus that causes AIDS.

Rocky Mountain News, Denver, April 15, 1994

"Dennis, is it possible for the state not to tell you where your mother is buried?" Jeanne almost shouts. [Dennis] Costa is used to meetings at which children cry for attention, and conversation swerves from school to a mother's grave. These are 12-year-olds, almost teenagers. They are dealing with changing bodies, changing emotions and changing lives. And their parents have died of AIDS. . . . "I'd like to see her on Mother's Day," Jeanne says wearily of her mother, whose grave she can't find. "I want to bring her flowers and I don't even know where she's at." This past May was Jeanne's first Mother's Day without her mom. Both her parents died of AIDS, two weeks apart.

The Plain Dealer, Cleveland, November 24, 1992.

AIDS breaks the rules of dying. It strikes predominantly the young, not the old. It decimates families and communities in a relentless onslaught of loss that allows but brief time to grieve one death before being confronted by another. Its continuing stigma produces silent grievers, like the forgotten children and youths who watch helplessly as death sweeps through their families.

How many of these children are there? No one knows, and no one is really counting. Instead of data we have projections, and they are likely underestimates. But because AIDS has become the leading cause of death for men in the child-rearing years and is rapidly approaching that status for women as well, the trajectory of this epidemic of childhood loss is clear: soon more children in the United States will lose parents to AIDS than to *any other* cause of death. Only a cure for HIV disease or a certain way to prevent its spread can alter this course. Neither is likely in the foreseeable future.

What *are* the projections? Michaels and Levine in 1992 estimated that by the year 2000 the number of children and adolescents in the United States left motherless because of AIDS would reach 72,000–125,000. Estimates by the United States Centers for Disease Control and Prevention are higher: during this decade, infected women will leave behind 125,000–150,000 children, about three-quarters of them uninfected. These projections, which CDC considers conservative, assume no increase in new HIV infections among women. Sadly, we already know that to be incorrect: new infections among women are climbing quickly and in all parts of the country.

Because these estimates focus on AIDS-related deaths of mothers only, they fail to account for many other AIDS-related losses that children and youths are experiencing. Deaths of fathers, sisters, brothers, of aunts and uncles, neighborhood friends, of teachers and classmates remain invisible in our current calculus of the impact of AIDS on our children.

Children whose lives are touched by AIDS confront not one epidemic but two. As the disease spreads, so does the epidemic of indifference to the children's plight. This book assumes that the epidemic of indifference, like the epidemic of AIDS, arises in part from ignorance—about the "disease" and about how to curb its impact. Through this book, we seek to arrest the epidemic of indifference by breaking society's silence about the children who must struggle to survive AIDS in their families.

The first seven chapters describe the wide array of challenges that AIDS presents to these forgotten children and youths. Chapter 1 describes trends and changes in the epidemic in the United States that pertain particularly to children and youths. Chapters 2 through 4 examine the psychological and emotional impact that a parent's or sibling's HIV disease has on uninfected children. The description in Chapter 2 of the medical aspects of AIDS suggests the "kaleidoscopic array of changes" that these children will witness in their homes as their parents and siblings become ill and die. Chapter 3 focuses on the significant impact of these many AIDS-related stresses on the uninfected child's normal development, and on the child's inability to master normal developmental tasks because of these stresses. Chapter 4 discusses more fully three of the AIDS-related stresses that pose particularly difficult problems for families living with AIDS: uncertainty, stigma, and secrecy. Because the adolescent survivors of AIDS in the family face special challenges, most notably the higher risk of becoming HIV-infected as well, Chapter 5 focuses on this population. Chapter 6 acknowledges that HIV infections occur in all cultures and among persons of all ethnicities, and discusses the need to develop culturally sensitive responses that respect differences in concepts of family responsibility, sickness, death, and grieving. Chapter 7 presents the many similarities—and the several notable differences—between children whose lives are torn by war and those who are suffering comparably traumatic losses because of AIDS.

The final five chapters frame a set of possible responses to these dual epidemics. Chapter 8 focuses on the extremely difficult and often painful questions that surround the inevitable change in custody from a dying parent to a "new" family and home. Chapter 9 outlines the current state of the law and suggests ways it might better respond, in three areas of particular moment: reducing the stigma surrounding AIDS, facilitating transitions in care and custody, and protecting the health of the surviving children and youths. Chapter 10 explores the significance of an African maxim, "It takes a village to raise a child," for children orphaned by this epidemic. It pushes us to reframe the context in which we think about this issue, and outlines in substantial detail the challenges posed to the child welfare, educational, child mental health, and legal systems, and to our community organizations and faith communities. Chapter 11 looks to the future, challenging us to think ahead and to begin debate on some of the hard questions that will too soon confront us. What happens when the present generation of grandmother-caretakers also dies? Will we see a resurgence of orphanages? Can we avoid transracial placements? Should we try to? Finally, Chapter 12 provides an agenda for action.

Throughout this book, three core themes emerge. The first concerns the challenges that HIV disease presents to these children: the profoundly disturbing physical and emotional deterioration that it causes in their parents and siblings; the disruptions, uncertainty, and unpredictability that scramble their young lives; the wrenching separations and multiple losses that it inflicts; and the silence and secrecy that it still commands. The second set of themes pertains to the children's response to this stigmatizing disease: their sense of personal responsibility for the well-being of their relatives—and, sometimes, even for the occurrence of the illness itself; their sense of isolation, vulnerability, and grief; their resilience when supported by others, and their troubling behavior when they are not. The third set of themes concerns the obligation of society to respond more appropriately to these children: to challenge our child welfare, mental health, legal, faith, and juvenile justice communities to meet their needs; to provide care for their burdened caretakers; and to combat AIDS-related stigma and discrimination so these children and their families need not suffer their great losses in silence.

Indeed, in asking us to confront this epidemic of indifference and to put

Part One

Voices:
A Mother and Two Children

Kara

Kara, extremely ill from AIDS, is sole parent to an uninfected six-year-old girl.

The reason I have to disguise myself is I'm concerned that my child, who does not have AIDS, won't be allowed to have friends at school or visit her friends' houses or have her friends visit her house. I'm afraid she'll be called names or teased. I have to hide my face because I have a terminal illness that everybody's afraid of, and my child would pay for it. She is paying for it. She's in pain. She lives it. She breathes it. She goes to bed with it every night.

Some nights we talk about it. Some nights she says, "Mommy, you'll be the Nana of my children, won't you?" And I say, "I hope so." And the next night she says, "Mommy, why can't the doctors make you better?" And the next night she says, "You won't be there, will you?" And the next night she'll say, "Who will take care of me?"

So she knows this, every day, every minute. Every time we used to say good-bye, she was afraid I might die then and there. We talked about that we'll know. She's seen me very sick. She's seen me eighty pounds. She's seen me almost die a few times. She's been rejected by every member of my family. She's been rejected by her father. She doesn't see him at all.

I guess the point here is that this is a child. I have to hide, she has to hide. I don't know how any human being can have any peace of mind hiding and deal with the loss of the only loved one you have.

I think any mother out there, if they take a look at their child and hold them in their arms . . . that's exactly how any woman with AIDS, with anything, feels about their child. And if any mother out there can look at their little child's little hands and know in two years they won't be there anymore . . . that's how I feel. That's how every woman feels with AIDS.

Me on the Outside, Me on the Inside

The illustrations labeled *Me on the Outside* and *Me on the Inside* were drawn by a ten-and-one-half-year-old girl whose mother and stepfather are HIV infected. In her "me on the outside picture" she portrays herself vacuuming, consistent with the caregiver role that she has assumed in the household. Because of her mother's hospitalizations and alcoholism, the girl has taken on the responsibility for household chores and the care of her younger sibling.

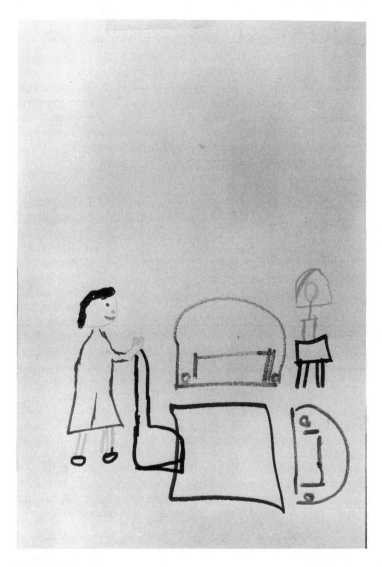

Me on the Outside

The girl's "me on the inside picture"—in which she portrays herself lying face down on her bed—captures her silent pain. Last year she told her best friend about her situation, hoping for some support. Some weeks later, as an act of revenge, the friend told the other children in the class that the girl's parents had AIDS. Suddenly teased and harassed by her peers, the girl felt forced to deny that her parents were infected. The harassment continued. To escape it, last year the girl and her family moved to a new community that does not know their family secret.

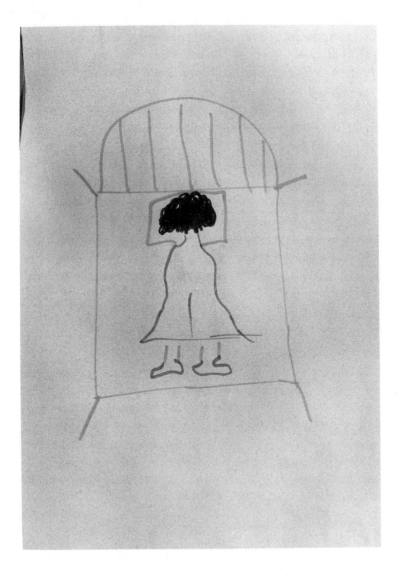

Me on the Inside

Onivea's Journal

"My mother died of AIDS, but I'm not ashamed of it. She was a nice person, and I loved her." Youngest of three children, Onivea began writing this series of letters addressed to her mother and God when she was ten years old. Her father had died when she was eight years old. A year later, when her mother died, Onivea moved into the home of a maternal aunt. She was "sad and mad," she explains, but adds, "I let out my feelings and I feel better. If I feel bad and I don't do anything, then I get an attitude." Onivea participates in a bereavement group organized by a local mental health agency. Started in 1988, the group helps Onivea and other children, sometimes as young as seven years old, resolve their grief about losing parents to AIDS. Onivea now is entering the turbulence of adolescence. She lives with a paternal aunt and is getting closer to her father's side of the family. Onivea takes great pride in her writing and in being able to help other children. She shares the following journal entries with you:

Dear God   3/8/92

You knew I, loved my mother
and how much we were
happy and that she had Adios
and her suffring but why
did you have to let her
die she was part of my
life now I feel bad becaus
she is no longer here to love me
anymore you took her away
from me and I will never
forgive you she was my
mother but you took her
from me she proble don'l
even i know me because she
is having a great time
in hevean I feel bad.
ps. I will forgive you because
I love you and you did that for a reasn
so she can be happy and because
and I also forgive you is becaus
you are my father

Love Onivea
Nicole Cruz

love you
mom and
God

3/12/92

Dear mom,

I love you so much and I miss you very much. I know you were fighting to live because you were worried about us... that we would go to a home or something but when Jenny told you not to worry that every thing is going to be all right because we could all live here they said that you had a big smile and I guest since you found out we will live here safe and happy We are happy here and I want to stay here but sometimes I just get selius because I see other kids with there mother and they always laughing and plaing and I can not do that any more because you are gone and I miss you If only I can touch or kiss or even hug you just once more I will be happy very happy

From Onivea Cruz

Dear mom,   3/22/9?

Yesterday Kesha was cring
because she missed you
I want to cry two but
what I really wanted to
do was to Show you that
I am strong and I can
hold the pain inside oi
me I love you and I will
always cry for you because
we belong together and
we are not together I
know you were strong to
fight that bad diease
but It is not fair I got
to see you once I saw
you you were ok and
the next day I finded
you dead that is not
right. I am so mad I can
not write nomore, for
now so by/.

♡ You

Dear mom,   3/30/9?

Hi there mom how are you
ding I am fine I hate to
Just write to you I like
to see you to talk to you face to
face You know Do You want to
know. Something sometimes
I think I killed you becaus
you would of never dieded
If I was not born If
only we had a second
chance I can make our
life better for us me
because I will be happy and
I would have a mother again
you because you would be happy
with your family and with
Robert and you three gen/s
mommy I love you by
now

you mommy

Dear mom   4/19/92

Hi there mom how are you
today I am fine You know
something mom I feel
empty without you and I
hate that feeling I would
like to feel full I would
like to have a mother in
my life at lease a mother
mommy I miss you so much
that day at the furnel I
just looked at you and I
saw someone In the coffen
I was saying to my self that
can't be mommy mommy is still
In the Hopistal It can't be
you I was so shocked. I
knew people had to die but I
never though about you dieing
you know I just felt you
holding me while I was crying
I just kept on saying It can
be you You Do not know how
hard It is to lose a beautyful
kind mother like you I got to
go.

by the way happy Easter
YOU   Love onivea

Dear mom   5/16/92

Hi mom I am Sorry I
Did'nt write to you for a
long time but I had a lot of
things on my mind and all those
things on my mind is my love
for you but you know
Something I thank Grandma
did a great job making you
and you did a great job
makeing all three of us
we all love you and we
know that you love us we
are a family but you
died even Though you are
dead we are still a family
and we will always willbe
a family well mom got to
go so by take one aunt and that makes us 4

Oniver   mom   Rosie   Kesha   Robert

Dear Anna mateo
By we love you

Macry

Part Two

The Challenge of AIDS to Children and Youth

Chapter 1

A Pandemic Out of Control
The Epidemiology of AIDS

BRIAN W. C. FORSYTH

In the first reports in 1981 of what appeared to be a new disease killing homosexual men and intravenous drug users, there was little indication of the enormity of what was to come. Within less than a decade the disease that is now called acquired immunodeficiency syndrome (AIDS) was to affect millions of people worldwide and to spread in the United States beyond the risk groups in which it was first described. It now affects people in all segments of the population, including ever-increasing numbers of women, children, and adolescents.

The virus that causes AIDS, now called the human immunodeficiency virus (HIV), was first isolated in 1984. The virus is transmitted either through sexual contact with someone who is infected or from receiving infected blood. A child whose mother is infected when she becomes pregnant or acquires the infection during pregnancy can be born with HIV. Although homosexual activity accounted for most sexually transmitted cases in the early years of the epidemic in the United States, heterosexual transmission is rapidly increasing. Blood-borne transmission has resulted in infection in three main groups: (*a*) intravenous drug users who exchange small amounts of infected blood when sharing needles; (*b*) people who received transfusions of infected blood or blood products—like clotting factors for the treatment of hemophilia—in the early years of the epidemic, before stringent testing for HIV was the rule; and (*c*) health care workers who have become infected as a result of accidents involving needles contaminated with infected blood.

Following infection with the virus a person may remain well for many years. In this stage of the disease, the individual is commonly described as HIV positive: a test to detect antibodies to the virus will be positive although there might be no other evidence of the disease. Eventually, the virus damages the immune system to such an extent that it can no longer provide defense against other infections; in addition, the normal regulatory processes that prevent tumors from developing are destroyed. The virus may also directly affect the brain and other organ systems. The term AIDS describes the stage at which certain characteristic manifestations of HIV disease become present, including specific infections or tumors, eventually leading to the individual's death.

Trends and Changes in the Epidemic

By the end of 1993, 361,509 cases of AIDS in the United States had been reported to the Centers for Disease Control and Prevention (CDC). As shown in Figure 1.1, the numbers of cases are occurring at an ever increasing rate—the first 100,000 cases occurred over an eight-year period, the second 100,000 were reported in only two and one-quarter years, and the third 100,000 in less than one and one-half years. The dramatic increase in 1993 resulted in part from an expansion in the case-reporting definition of AIDS to include HIV-positive individuals who, though not seriously ill, show evidence of severely damaged immune systems (that is, a low CD4+ lymphocyte count).

The statistics on reported cases of AIDS, however, fail to portray the true extent of the epidemic. There is no national system for reporting persons who are HIV infected but who do not yet have AIDS (although more than half of the fifty states now require named HIV reporting, and CDC will include HIV reports in future surveillance reports). Because of the long delay between infection and the development of AIDS, statistics on reported cases reflect patterns of infection occurring seven to ten years ago. Estimates in 1994 are that approximately one million persons in the United States are infected with the virus—1 in every 250. Approximately twenty thousand of these are children. On a global scale, the World Health Organization has estimated that thirteen million adults and one million children are infected.[1]

In the early years of the epidemic in this country, persons infected with the virus were predominantly white homosexual or bisexual males or intravenous drug users. In recent years, however, there has been a significant change in the characteristics of the epidemic. Table 1.1 compares cases reported in 1992 with those reported in the previous year. (Statistics from 1993 are not used because the change in the case definition that occurred in that year distorts comparisons with previous years.) Although males still account for the large majority of cases, the proportional increase for females is significantly greater. Similarly, although infections among homosexual or bisexual men still account for about half of the cases, the number of cases actually decreased slightly between these two years. By comparison, cases involving injecting drug users increased slightly, and heterosexual transmission accounted for the largest proportional increase.

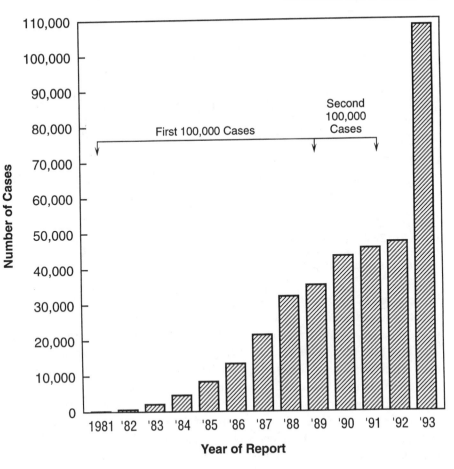

Figure 1.1. Reported cases of AIDS in the United States by year. Source: Based on Centers for Disease Control and Prevention, 1992, The second 100,000 cases of acquired immunodeficiency syndrome—United States, June 1981–December 1991, *Morbidity and Mortality Weekly Report* 41 (2): 28–29, and 1992–93 surveillance data provided by Centers for Disease Control and Prevention, Public Health Service, United States Department of Health and Human Services.

The epidemic is also increasingly affecting ethnic minorities and women. In 1992, 34 percent of those reported as having AIDS were African-American and 17 percent were Hispanic, whereas in the first five years of the epidemic 25 percent were African-American and 14 percent Hispanic. Similarly, in 1992, 13 percent of cases involved women, compared with only 7 percent of the cases reported in the first five years of the epidemic. This trend is even more prominent in particular areas of the country. For example, women accounted for 22 percent of the cases reported in New York State between 1991 and 1993; in some cities more than a third of the cases are women. Younger women are

Table 1.1   Comparison of AIDS Cases Reported in 1991 and 1992

| | Number of Reported Cases of AIDS | | Percentage Change |
	1991	1992	
Males	39,100	40,080	+2.5%
Females	5,732	6,255	+9.1%
Homosexual & Bisexual Males	24,216	23,936	-1.2%
Injecting Drug Users	11,314	11,425	+1.0%
Heterosexual Contact	3,512	4,114	+17.1%
Total adult/adolescent	44,832	46,335	+3.4%

Source: Based on data provided by the Centers for Disease Control and Prevention, Public Health Service, United States Department of Health and Human Services in *HIV/AIDS Surveillance Reports* for 1991, 1992.

being affected at a disproportionate rate: in 1991, 27 percent of the fifteen- to twenty-four-year-old age group reported with AIDS were women, whereas for the group aged twenty-five to forty-four years, only 12 percent were women.

There have also been important changes in the geographic distribution of cases within the United States. In the early years of the epidemic, cases were clustered in large urban areas, in particular in New York City and San Francisco. Although there continues to be a preponderance of cases in large cities, the number of cases in smaller cities and rural areas has increased. As illustrated in Figure 1.2, the epidemic is no longer limited to a few regions: a majority of the states now report significant numbers of cases.

Studies designed to determine the prevalence of HIV infection among women giving birth have provided further information on the extent of the epidemic among women and children. Such studies have used a technique for detecting HIV antibodies in blood specimens that are routinely obtained to screen newborn babies for genetic disorders. These studies have demonstrated dramatic differences in infection rates among women in different parts of the United States and among different ethnic groups. States on the eastern seaboard have rates many times greater than elsewhere in the country. New York State has the highest rate of infection: in a study done in 1989, approximately 1 in every 150 women giving birth was infected (and in parts of New York City the figure reached 1 in 45). The rate of infection was many times higher for African-American and Hispanic women (1.8 percent and 1.3 percent, respectively) than for white women (0.13 percent).

The changes in the epidemic over time are due to a number of factors. There is evidence, for example, that educational efforts directed toward homosexual men have resulted in some changes in behavior that have pro-

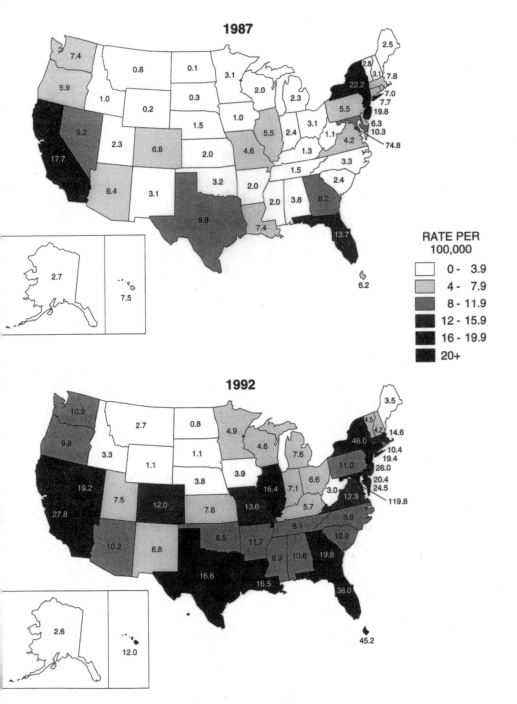

Figure 1.2. A comparison of annual rates of AIDS per 100,000 population for cases reported in 1987 and 1992. Source: Based on data provided by the Centers for Disease Control and Prevention, Public Health Service, United States Department of Health and Human Services in *HIV/AIDS Surveillance Reports* for 1987, 1992.

duced a lower rate of infection. This is more pronounced among older homosexual men than among young ones, however, and educational efforts among other groups, such as intravenous drug users, appear to have been less successful. New infections from contaminated blood or blood products are now virtually nonexistent because all donated blood is now tested for the virus. The changes in the AIDS epidemic mimic the course of other epidemics: infections quickly spread through the population groups who are first affected or those who are most at risk. Then, as the initial spread declines in these groups, a more gradual increase in infection affects others who were initially less at risk. In the United States transmission among heterosexual partners represents the second wave of the epidemic. Between 1991 and 1992 heterosexual transmission accounted for the largest proportionate increase in reported AIDS cases, and in 1993 there was a 130 percent increase in the number of cases due to heterosexual transmission over the previous year.

AIDS as a Leading Cause of Death

As AIDS has become increasingly prevalent it has emerged as a leading cause of death, causing increasing numbers of children to be affected through the loss of their parents and other family members. By the end of 1993, 220,871 persons in the United States had lost their lives to this disease—more than four times the number of Americans who died in the Vietnam War. As dramatic as these figures are, they are almost certainly an underestimate: AIDS is not identified as the cause of death in about one quarter of the deaths that are HIV-related.[2]

The epidemic has affected young adults disproportionately. In 1992 it became the leading cause of death in the United States for men between the ages of twenty-five and forty-four years (see Figure 1.3). It is already the fourth-leading cause of death of young women, and current trends suggest that it will eventually become the leading cause for that group as well (see Figure 1.4). Already, more children in this country lose their mothers each year to AIDS than to automobile accidents. By 1990, AIDS was the number one cause of death of young women in nine large cities in the country. Also, because ethnic minority populations are disproportionately affected by AIDS, the disease accounts for a greater proportion of deaths among these groups. The death rate from AIDS for young African-American men is about three times that of young white men. The differences for women are even greater: the death rate from AIDS among African-American women is about twelve times that of white women. Although AIDS was only the fourth-leading cause of death of all women between the ages of twenty-five and forty-four in 1992, it was the second-leading cause of death among African-American women and the third-leading cause of death among Hispanic women.

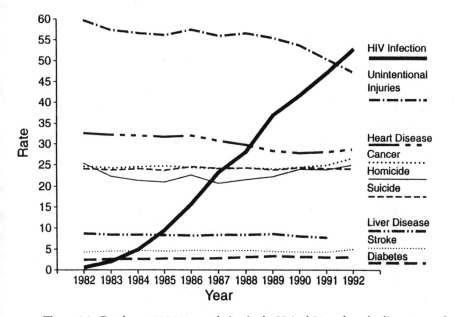

Figure 1.3. Deaths per 100,000 population in the United States from leading causes of death among men ages 25–44 years. Source: Centers for Disease Control and Prevention, 1993, Update: Mortality attributable to HIV infection among persons aged 25–44 Years—United States, 1991 and 1992, *Morbidity and Mortality Weekly Report* 42 (45): 869–872.

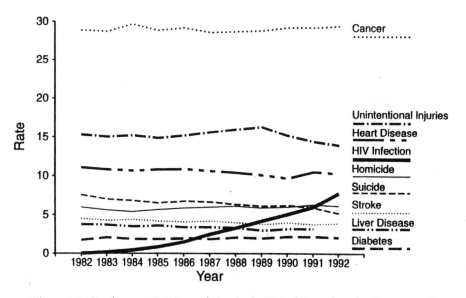

Figure 1.4. Deaths per 100,000 population in the United States from leading causes of death among women ages 25–44 years. Source: see Figure 1.3.

Children with HIV Infection

AIDS was first described in children in 1982, only one year after it had been described in adults. By the end of 1993, there had been 5,234 cases of AIDS reported in children under the age of thirteen years. At the start of the epidemic, a large proportion of these cases involved children who had received transfusions of contaminated blood or blood products, but such cases account for only a minority of the cases in more recent years. Ninety-three percent of the cases among children reported in 1993 were due to mother-to-child transmission of the virus. It is now known that transmission can occur either during the pregnancy, at birth, or postnatally as a result of breast-feeding. Fortunately, a minority of babies born to infected mothers are themselves infected, between 13 and 33 percent, according to various studies. Whether infected or not, all babies born to infected mothers will initially have a positive HIV antibody test, reflecting the presence of maternal antibodies.

Children with AIDS are predominantly African-American and Hispanic. Of the child AIDS cases reported in 1993, these two groups accounted for 55 percent and 27 percent, respectively.

Unlike adults with HIV infection who often remain asymptomatic for many years, infected children tend to become symptomatic very quickly. Approximately 70 percent develop symptoms by one year of age and about 17 percent die within the first year. AIDS is now a leading cause of death of children in the one-to-four-year age group. In 1990 it became the leading cause of death among Hispanic children in this age group and the second-leading cause of death among African-American children of the same age. However, over half of the children who are infected live to seven years of age, and some children who were born in the early years of the epidemic are now adolescents.

HIV and Adolescents

Compared with other age groups, the number of adolescents reported with AIDS is relatively small. By the end of 1993, there had been 1,528 reported cases in the United States among persons between the ages of thirteen and nineteen years. These figures underestimate the severity of the problem of HIV disease among adolescents, however, and tend to minimize the potential future impact of this disease on them. Because it often takes a number of years after infection before a person develops AIDS-defining symptoms, individuals who are infected as adolescents often do not develop symptoms until their twenties and therefore are not included in the "teenage" AIDS statistics. Approximately one-fifth of cases of AIDS are diagnosed in individuals aged between twenty and twenty-nine years. A large proportion of these individuals likely acquired their infection during their adolescent years. In addition, in 1993 there was a greater proportionate increase in reported cases among the thirteen-to-twenty-four-year age group than among all other ages.

Studies designed to assess the prevalence of HIV infection, rather than only those with the AIDS diagnosis, are helpful in estimating the true extent of infection among adolescents. Studies of college students, for example, have shown an overall rate of infection of 0.2 percent—that is, approximately 1 in 500 of the students tested was infected. Among Job Corps applicants, who are more likely to come from more disadvantaged backgrounds, data collected between 1987 and 1990 showed that 1 in every 278 applicants was infected. Much higher rates were found in certain geographic areas and among certain races. For example, in urban areas in the Northeast, 1 in 40 African-American and Hispanic twenty-one-year-old Job Corps applicants was infected.[3] An alarming finding comes from studies over two different time periods in an adolescent health clinic in Washington, D.C. When all adolescents attending the clinic were screened in 1987, 1 in every 244 was found to be infected. Five years later the rate of infection in the same clinic was almost five times as great: 1 in 52.[4]

Among adolescents there is not the same discrepancy in rates of infection between males and females as exists in adults. In fact, there has been a change over time, and in some populations the infection rate is now greater among young adolescent females than in males of the same age. Among the reasons for this phenomenon is the important role that heterosexual sex plays in transmission among adolescents; furthermore, in heterosexual sex the virus is more easily transmitted from male to female than vice versa. The increasing rate of infection among young women will, in turn, lead to an increase in the number of children born to infected mothers.

Patterns of behavior among adolescents and the difficulties inherent in trying to decrease their high-risk behaviors suggest that the infection rate in that age group will almost certainly increase. According to the results of the 1990 Youth Risk Behavior Survey, a large national survey of high school students, approximately one-third of females and one-half of males report having had sexual intercourse by ninth grade; at the same time, fewer than half of sexually active adolescents reported using a condom when they last had sexual intercourse.[5] Statistics on such other sexually transmitted diseases as gonorrhea and syphilis confirm that young people are at risk. Nearly two-thirds of the more than twelve million cases of sexually transmitted diseases reported nationally in 1990 were among persons under the age of twenty-five. Every year, one of every eight sexually active adolescents is infected with a sexually transmitted disease. These statistics suggest that large numbers of adolescents are failing to protect themselves against sexually transmitted diseases, the most serious of which is AIDS. In addition, there is evidence that the presence of open lesions from other sexually transmitted diseases facilitates transmission of HIV, putting the individual at even greater risk of contracting the infection.

Adolescents frequently experiment with alcohol and drugs. Although intravenous drugs account for only a small proportion of this drug use (approximately 2 percent of high school students), the use of other drugs and alcohol can lead to impaired judgment, which can in turn promote unsafe sexual practices. Statistics from the 1990 Youth Risk Behavior Survey indicated that 30 percent of female high school students and 44 percent of male students had taken five or more drinks on at least one occasion in the prior month.

Some evidence suggests that increased educational efforts have brought about some changes in sexual behavior among adolescents. National surveys of high school students between 1989 and 1991 show that the percentage reporting that they had ever had sexual intercourse dropped from 59 percent to 54 percent, and the numbers reporting multiple sex partners also decreased.[6] Over the same time period, the proportion of students reporting that they had received HIV instruction in school increased from 54 percent to 83 percent. Although there was little change in condom use among the whole student population (46 percent in 1990 to 48 percent in 1991), sexually active students under fifteen years of age reported an increase in condom use from 46 percent to 57 percent. This supports the notion that educational efforts may have a greater impact on changing the behaviors of younger adolescents who are not yet sexually active or are just becoming sexually active than of those who have been sexually active for some time. Although these statistics show some promise, there needs to be significantly more change in order to avoid a major epidemic of HIV disease among adolescents.

Children's Experience of HIV Among Family and Friends

It is estimated that approximately forty-five thousand children and adolescents in this country will have been "orphaned" as a result of the AIDS epidemic by the end of 1995; as shown in Figure 1.5, this number is expected to rise to as many as 125,000 by the end of this decade.[7] The term *orphan* as used in these estimates refers to the death of a child's mother only. These projections were extrapolated from the death rates of women with AIDS. They likely underestimate the number of children who will be left motherless because the model assumes that annual AIDS-related deaths among women will plateau at their projected 1993 number. Recent data suggest, however, that the number of such deaths continues to increase. Approximately three-quarters of women with HIV infection have children.[8] The majority of them are unmarried and therefore have primary responsibility for the care of their children.

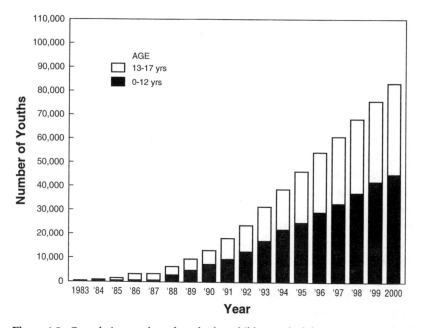

Figure 1.5. Cumulative number of motherless children and adolescents estimated to be orphaned by the AIDS epidemic in the United States. Source: D. Michaels and C. Levine, 1992, Estimates of the number of motherless youth orphaned by AIDS in the United States, *Journal of the American Medical Association* 268: 3456–3461. Copyright © 1992, AMA.

Clearly, however, the picture of the impact of AIDS on children is much more complicated. We have little understanding of the extent to which children are experiencing the illnesses and deaths of their fathers and other loved ones. Similarly, we know little about who looks after these children once they lose their parents or even before their parents die. One study examined who was caring for children who had been born to infected mothers.[9] These were children enrolled in a study in six regions of the country through the end of 1990. Only 56 percent of the children were living with a biologic parent; 27 percent were living in foster homes, 10 percent with relatives, 3 percent with adoptive parents, and 4 percent in group settings or with other caregivers. This distribution was not significantly different whether or not the child was infected. There were some geographic differences. In New York City, for example, only 42 percent of children were living with a biologic parent as compared with Texas, where 70 percent were. Only 6.3 percent of mothers in the study were known to be deceased, and maternal intravenous drug use was the most important factor associated with children living with alternative caregivers. But this study was only one view of an evolving situation: as time goes on, more parents will die. Infected children may die before their parents, but those who outlive their parents—and the many more uninfected children who experience the deaths of their parents—will continue to need nurturing care.

What Does the Future Hold?

Although there have been advances in the treatment of HIV-related disease, no treatment yet has halted or even slowed the tremendous expansion of the epidemic. It is difficult to provide accurate long-term projections of the numbers that will be infected in the future, but it seems almost certain that the spread of the infection will plateau in the group that currently accounts for the larger number already infected—homosexual men—while the spread will increase steadily among people acquiring the infection through intravenous drug use and heterosexual transmission. Thus the proportion of cases occurring among women, children, and adolescents will continue to increase. Because infection is already more prevalent among minority populations in large urban centers, the epidemic will also almost certainly expand disproportionately among these groups, and the current differences in the degrees to which people in different racial and socioeconomic groups are affected will be magnified.

Thus the epidemiology of HIV in the United States will tend to become more like that in other parts of the world, where heterosexual transmission is already the major cause for spread of the infection. In sub-Saharan Africa, for example, infected women already outnumber men by a ratio of six to five. The World Health Organization estimates that already over half of all infections in the world are in persons between the ages of fifteen and twenty-four. By the year 2000 it is estimated that there will be thirty million to forty million people infected worldwide. Of these, approximately thirteen million will be women, and there will be between five and ten million orphaned children.

Notes

1. United Nations Children's Fund (UNICEF), 1993, *AIDS: The second decade—a focus on youth and women,* New York: UNICEF.

2. Buehler, J. W., et al., 1990, Impact of the human immunodeficiency virus epidemic on mortality trends in young men, United States, *American Journal of Public Health* 80: 1080–1086.

3. St. Louis, M., et al., 1991, Human immunodeficiency virus infection in disadvantaged adolescents: Findings from the US Job Corps, *Journal of the American Medical Association* 266 (17): 2387–2391.

4. D'Angelo, L. J., 1994, HIV infection and AIDS in adolescents, in *Pediatric AIDS: The challenge of HIV infection in infants, children and adolescents,* 2d ed., ed. P. A. Pizzo and C. M. Wilfert, 71–81. Baltimore: Williams & Wilkins.

5. Centers for Disease Control, 1992, Sexual behavior among high school students—United States, 1990, *Morbidity and Mortality Weekly Reports* 40: 885–888.

6. Centers for Disease Control, 1992, HIV instruction and selected HIV-risk behaviors

among high school students—United States, 1989–1991, *Morbidity and Mortality Weekly Reports* 41 (46): 866–868.

7. Michaels, D., and C. Levine, 1992, Estimates of the number of motherless youth orphaned by AIDS in the United States, *Journal of the American Medical Association* 268: 3456–3461.

8. Niebuhr, V., J. Hughes, and R. Pollard, 1994, Parents with human immunodeficiency virus infection: Perceptions of their children's emotional needs, *Pediatrics* 93 (3): 421–42.

9. Caldwell, M. B., et al., 1992, Biologic, foster and adoptive parents: Care givers of children exposed perinatally to human immunodeficiency virus in the United States, *Pediatrics* 90 (4): 603–607.

Chapter 2

Medical Aspects of AIDS
What Do Children Witness?

WARREN ANDIMAN

Uninfected children in AIDS-affected families witness a kaleido-scopic array of changes in their homes. As the disease progresses, those infected often undergo profound physical and emotional alterations. The provision of care brings about many other changes in the home. Travel between home, hospital, clinic, and social service agencies disrupts the daily routines of the family and further saps the energies of persons already enervated by the disease.

Much care of HIV-affected families occurs within a traditional medical context. Therefore, in this chapter I will summarize current concepts concerning mother-to-child transmission of HIV and the natural history of the infection. I will also describe the major clinical manifestations of HIV infection as they occur in both children and adults, and I will review recent data concerning prognosis and survival. Finally, I will attempt to paint a picture that describes the somewhat fractious imposition of new objects, new routines (AIDS clinical trials, for example), and new people within the lives of these families, and I will demonstrate how these changes are likely to increase the level of confusion in already chaotic lives.

Background: Vertical Transmission and Natural History

Two basic concepts about HIV infection and AIDS govern our understanding of how the disease is perceived within the context of a household that includes at least one infected adult, usually a mother. First, only a minority of children born to infected women are infected themselves. Second, the natural history of the infection varies greatly from individual to individual, and the manifestations of disease, when they occur, are protean. These two circumstances conspire to create an environment characterized by unpredictability. An HIV-seropositive woman cannot know during her pregnancy or for at least several months following the birth of her baby whether the child is infected or not. Furthermore, when more than one person with HIV infection resides in the same home, no one can accurately predict the order in which they will get sick, nor the specific incarnations the disease will take in those infected. The course of the infection is just as unpredictable in adults as in children.

Mother-to-Child Transmission of HIV

In the industrialized countries of the world, the rate of vertical (mother-to-child) transmission of HIV varies from 13 to 33 percent.[1] These rates are derived from prospective, longitudinal cohort studies conducted in Europe and the United States in which investigators have been able to clearly distinguish the subgroup of infected children from those who are uninfected by using some combination of virologic, serologic, and molecular biologic techniques. These data indicate that the great majority of children—approximately 65–85 percent—born to infected mothers are *not* themselves infected. It has been more difficult to derive accurate rates of mother-to-child transmission of HIV in Africa or Asia, but for reasons that are unclear, they appear to be higher than in the developed countries of the world.[2] The higher incidence of other untreated sexually transmitted diseases in these parts of the world may contribute to the higher rates of transmission of HIV to the fetus. In addition, there may be methodologic problems and deficiencies in surveillance that contribute to this discrepancy.

It is important to remember that, infected or not, *all* HIV-*exposed* children have infected mothers. Many live in households that might also include others who are infected: fathers, siblings, other first-degree relatives, close friends, or, on rare occasions, grandparents.

Much research has been done in an effort to identify specific maternal risk factors associated with vertical transmission of the virus. Advanced maternal disease, a low CD4+ cell count (see Glossary, p. 48), a low CD4+:CD8+ cell ratio, and the presence of the virus and viral-associated proteins in blood have generally been accepted as variables associated with transmission of virus to the infant.[3] There is also accumulating evidence that vaginal delivery is associated with greater risk of vertical transmission than Caesarean section.[4] Current research is directed at determining: (*a*) whether the amount of virus present affects the likelihood of transmission; (*b*) whether specific variants of the virus with particular biologic or molecular properties are more apt to be transmitted than are others; and (*c*) whether there are particular components of the maternal or fetal immune responses to the virus (for example, neutralizing antibody, cytotoxic T cells) that influence the risk of vertical transmission.

It seems apparent that HIV can be transmitted at all stages of pregnancy and that a significant proportion of transmission events, perhaps 50 percent or more, occur at the time of delivery, when the infant is covered with virus-laden maternal blood and secretions.[5] Virus can also be transmitted by way of breast milk, although in the United States virtually all HIV-positive mothers favor formula feeding over breast-feeding.[6] The relative proportion of pediatric infections attributable to transmission during each stage of pregnancy and postpartum is yet to be determined, but defining these proportions is critical, because various interventions designed to interrupt transmission are applicable to one stage but not to others. Infections that occur early in pregnancy, for example, might be prevented by immunizing the mother with a protective or therapeutic vaccine before she becomes pregnant, as we do currently to prevent the congenital anomalies associated with rubella. Infections that are transmitted at the time of delivery, on the other hand, might be prevented by providing the baby with a hyperimmune globulin product, as well as the first in a series of protective vaccinations, within twenty-four hours of delivery. Such a strategy of providing both passive and active immunization to abort peripartum transmission of an infectious agent has been used with great success in the case of hepatitis B. Results of a multicenter trial in which zidovudine (AZT) was given to a specific subgroup of infected women during pregnancy and delivery and to their offspring postpartum point strongly to a protective effect of the drug in reducing the risk of vertical transmission— an effect probably attributable to a decrease in the mother's viral burden.

In some cases, babies presumed to have been infected with HIV in utero have been shown to be virus culture-positive in the first week of life; cultures of babies infected at delivery, by contrast, do not reveal the presence of virus until weeks or even months following delivery. Virus acquired by the baby at birth must go through multiple cycles of replication in order to reach a quantity that can be detected by culture or by the polymerase chain reaction.

Pathogenesis and Natural History of Infection

HIV has multiple cellular targets within humans. Although the effects of HIV on the immune system are, to a great extent, due to the direct and indirect damage it does to CD4+ T lymphocytes, the virus is capable of attaching to and infecting many other kinds of cells. These targets include cells in the skin and lymphoid tissues, bone marrow precursor cells, various kinds of cells in the central nervous system (most notably microglial cells), and cardiac muscle cells, as well as cells in the rectal mucosa, the uterine cervix, and the kidney. In most instances, infection of these cells is due to the presence on their surfaces of the CD4+ receptor, but there is now accumulating evidence that HIV can utilize a receptor other than CD4 or that two receptors, including CD4, may act in concert as an attachment site for the virus. In the peripheral blood, HIV has been identified in cells other than lymphocytes, especially in monocytes. Unlike CD4+ lymphocytes, which usually die following invasion by the virus, monocytic cells appear to survive infection and may be responsible for carrying infection to the lung and the brain. They may harbor the virus for long periods of time, in relative isolation from the actions of the immune system.

Although the virus is present in relatively small quantities in circulating blood cells, there is now ample evidence that the virus can be widely disseminated in lymphoid tissues of the body, beginning at the earliest stages of infection. Lymphoid organs may serve as the principal reservoir of virus in the body. The involvement of the developing thymus in this process among infected children, along with infection of progenitor cells in the bone marrow, may account for the profound hematologic and immunologic defects observed.

The temporal course and duration of HIV infection and AIDS vary greatly from one individual to the next, although, in general, the disease among adults is characterized by an unusually long clinical latency period—the interval between acute infection and the appearance of AIDS-associated signs. Death, too, follows AIDS at varying intervals. The median clinical latency period, during which patients are for the most part asymptomatic, ranges from seven to ten years.

In general, the duration of clinical latency and the interval between AIDS and death are shorter for HIV-infected children than for adults. Our estimates of the duration of life free of symptoms can be determined much more accurately for children, because infection is acquired by virtually all children in utero or at the time of delivery; hence the time of infection can be narrowed to a nine-month period.

New and experimental treatments may lengthen the period of clinical latency or may rearrange the order in which certain conditions occur. Successful prophylactic treatments for *Pneumocystis carinii* pneumonia have reduced the incidence among AIDS patients of this infection, which once killed many individuals in the early stages of the full-blown disease. Consequently, patients now are more likely to acquire other infections (for example, atypical mycobacterial infection) or other conditions (wasting disease, lymphoma) for which prophylactic or curative treatments have not yet been proven successful.

Among pediatric cases that are perinatally acquired, the median age at time of diagnosis of AIDS is approximately twelve months, though perhaps 1 to 2 percent of pediatric patients are not diagnosed with AIDS until ten years of age or later. Data collected from various institutions in the United States and Europe confirm observations made at Yale that suggest strongly a bimodal pattern in expression of disease and in survival.[7] Models describing survival among childhood populations indicate that approximately 10 to 15 percent of children are likely to die before age four years, with a median age at death of five to eleven months. Among those surviving beyond four years, the median age at death is more than sixty months.

These phenomena have an impact on what uninfected children in HIV-affected families may witness. For example, because the clinical latency period is foreshortened in many children when compared to that of their parents, uninfected children may see their siblings die before their parents even show signs of disease. Because some infected children survive, with symptoms, into early adolescence, their siblings may spend a decade or more living with a brother or sister who is getting progressively more debilitated.

Clinical Course of Infection in Children and Adults

What Do Uninfected Children See?

Because of great individual variation in the clinical latency period in both children and adults, uninfected children in affected households are likely to be confused by what they witness. Confusion is particularly likely if these uninfected children suspect, but have not been told, that their siblings, parents, aunts, or uncles have HIV infection. Believing that AIDS is rapidly fatal, they may expect their relatives to be immediately debilitated and dysfunctional. Instead, in many instances, they observe these infected persons going to work or to school and negotiating the business of their daily activities without apparent difficulty. These prolonged asymptomatic periods provide an important argument for those who desire to keep their condition a secret: Why alarm the uninfected child with the news that you or another member of your household is infected when you feel quite well and can easily accomplish the tasks of daily living? (Of course, the decision to maintain the secret does not come without a price, as we shall see in Chapter 4.) The long asymptomatic period may be punctuated, toward its end but before AIDS occurs, by subtle expressions of fatigue, periodic low-grade fevers, gastrointestinal upset, oral thrush, and lymph node enlargement. These signs of illness are often temporary and do not interfere with activity for more than a few days or weeks.

Clinical Presentations of HIV Disease in Children

Much of what we know about the frequency and natural history of AIDS-associated illnesses in HIV-positive children has been derived from prospective, longitudinal cohort studies of HIV-seropositive children who have been identified around the time of birth.[8] Other critical data are collected through both active and passive surveillance by state health departments and federal agencies.

Between 1982 and 1992 the Centers for Disease Control and Prevention collected data on the most common AIDS indicator diseases among children. They included, in rank order: *P. carinii* pneumonia (PCP) (affecting 37 percent of juvenile AIDS patients), lymphoid interstitial pneumonia (25 percent), recurrent bacterial infections (19 percent), wasting disease (14 percent), *Candida* esophagitis (13 percent) and HIV encephalopathy (12 percent). Cytomegalovirus disease, pulmonary candidiasis, atypical mycobacterium infection, cryptosporidiosis and diseases due to *Herpes simplex* each occurred in fewer than 10 percent of patients.

Cumulative data and clinical impressions arising from multiple medical centers point to two distinctive patterns of disease presentation and evolution of illness among infected children. One group of patients develops severe and progressive disease in infancy. Many of these patients have a constellation of AIDS-associated diseases, including some or all of the following: *P. carinii* pneumonia, cytomegalovirus disease, marked failure-to-thrive, and encephalopathy. Many of these "early presenters" die in the first year or two of life. The other group is composed of long-term survivors, many of whom do not develop HIV-associated conditions until age three or older. These conditions often include lymphoid interstitial pneumonitis (LIP), parotitis, diffuse swelling of lymphoid organs, recurrent otitis media and slowly progressive neurologic disease (sometimes manifest initially as subtle disorders of mental activity or as school failure). Disease progression in this latter group is more indolent. Eventually, most of the later presenters will develop illnesses that characterize their state of prolonged survival: chronic pulmonary disease with bronchiectasis, chronic sinusitis, disseminated atypical mycobacterial infection, lymphoma, and severe wasting disease. (These diseases may also occur, but less frequently, in the early presenters.) Static or progressive encephalopathy may also develop in these late survivors. Among children followed in New Haven, Connecticut, LIP is the singular disease that has occurred *only* among long-term survivors, in whom characteristic abnormalities in the chest X-ray first begin to appear in the second or third year of life.

In past surveys, PCP has occurred in as many as 60 percent of children diagnosed with AIDS in the first twelve months of life. Although early identification of infected infants, institution of prophylactic regimens for PCP, and more rapid diagnosis and treatment of overt PCP infection have improved overall survival among pediatric AIDS patients, PCP is still a cause of early and unexpected mortality in infants under six months of age. This frequently results from the absence of prior knowledge of the child's (and often the mother's) seropositive status before the onset of the acute illness. If HIV counseling and testing were more a routine part of women's health care, these unexpected pediatric illnesses would be largely eliminated, for those HIV-exposed babies who receive ongoing medical care and who are identified as being at special risk would receive prophylactic treatment for PCP.

In recent years, a variety of medications have been developed to prevent or to delay the progression of certain opportunistic pathogens. In addition, antiretroviral agents, such as zidovudine (AZT, ZDV), didanosine (ddI) and zalcitibine (ddC) have been used to treat the primary infection. More widespread use of combinations of these drugs is likely to change permanently the natural history of the disease, largely by delaying the occurrence of AIDS-defining illnesses and lengthening, by a year or two, the asymptomatic stage of infection.

Course and Outcome of Infection in Children

An Italian study of nearly 1,900 children born to HIV-seropositive mothers found that HIV-associated signs of disease developed in 82 percent of infected children at a median age of five months; these signs appeared earlier in those who subsequently died than in those who survived until the time of data analysis.[9] Of those identified at birth and followed continuously thereafter, 24 percent had died of AIDS at a median age of fourteen months, but half of those infected survived to age nine years.

In this cohort, three patterns of illness were described: (a) those with the mildest illness had a constellation of signs consisting of hepatosplenomegaly, lymph node enlargement, parotitis, skin diseases and recurrent respiratory infections; (b) those with an intermediate level of disease had lymphoid interstitial pneumonitis (LIP) and/or idiopathic thrombocytopenic purpura (ITP); and (c) those with the most severe pattern of disease had opportunistic infections, severe bacterial infections, progressive neurologic disease, anemia and recurrent unexplained fevers. By univariate analysis, the conditions associated with the worst prognosis included growth failure, persistent oral candidiasis, hepatitis and AIDS cardiopathy.

Recent studies conducted at Yale by Brian Forsyth et al. and B. Joyce Simpson et al. showed that 41 percent of children who were infected perinatally between 1979 and 1992 have died; three-quarters of these children succumbed to the disease before the age of three years. A clinical staging system was developed retrospectively in order to describe the association between certain clusters of signs of disease and survival. Among patients in the first year of life with encephalopathy and opportunistic infections (including PCP), or with persistent oral candidiasis, serious bacterial infections and persistent fevers, prognosis and survival were significantly poorer than among children with less severe degrees of illness (for example, hepatomegaly, failure-to-thrive). The median life span for infants who experienced neurologic disease or PCP by age nine months was only 1.1 years. In contrast, patients with the mildest forms of illness in the first year of life survived for a median of 9.6 years.

A prospective analysis of the outcomes among 229 children born to HIV-infected women since late 1985 revealed that 9.2 percent had developed AIDS during the first seven years of the study. Some patients developed multiple AIDS-defining illnesses (ADI); there were thirty-six such illnesses among the twenty-one patients with AIDS. *P. carinii* pneumonia was the most common ADI among those who died, and LIP was the most frequent among those who survived. Among those who died, the mean interval between first ADI and death was 9.6 months; between second ADI and death the mean interval was 6.5 months. Six of fourteen patients died within ninety days of their second ADI. These data indicate that once an AIDS-defining illness (other than LIP) occurs in a child, especially an infant, the family should be prepared for inexorable physical decline and the possibility of death in less than a year.

Course of Infection in Adults

As noted earlier, the symptom-free period in adults—the time between infection and clinical expression of disease—is much longer than for most infectious diseases, extending, as it does, nearly a decade in the majority of infected individuals (see Figure 2.1).[10] The onset of HIV-associated illness is heralded by a slow and inexorable decline in the CD4+ T lymphocyte count (to levels lower than two hundred cells per microliter), the reappearance of HIV proteins in blood, and, sometimes, by declining hemoglobin levels and platelet counts. Clinical predictors of progression to AIDS include a constellation of constitutional symptoms (for example, unexplained fever and weight loss), diarrhea, thrush and hairy leukoplakia (an Epstein-Barr virus–associated malady of the tongue). It is currently believed that all or nearly all HIV seropositive individuals will ultimately develop AIDS because, even in those persons who have remained asymptomatic for extended periods, evidence of immune deficiency can almost always be demonstrated by laboratory tests.

Involvement of a multiplicity of cells and tissue types in the pathologic process, sometimes from the earliest stages of infection, account for the protean manifestations of the disease. Epidemiologists and clinicians have described the relative frequency of the various clinical signs and diseases that constitute AIDS in populations of individuals affected by HIV. Although such studies can be used to prioritize treatment interventions or to develop care plans for the immediate future, they cannot be used with any degree of certainty in predicting the expression of the illness in a particular patient.

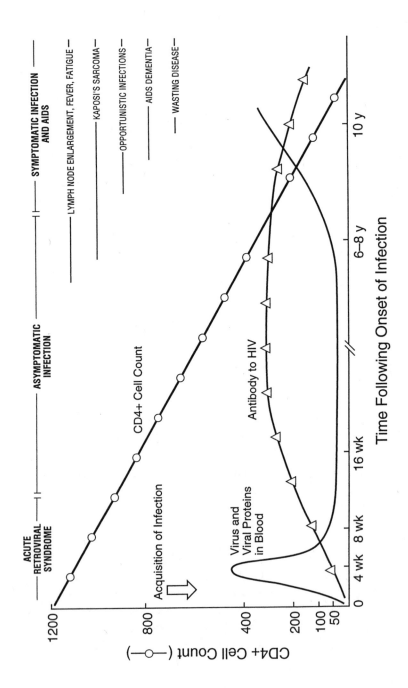

Figure 2.1. Course of HIV infection in adults.

When signs and symptoms finally appear, they include physical changes, behavioral and cognitive changes, and, often, severe debilitation and inanition. For any given patient it is impossible to predict how quickly the disease will progress to AIDS and, thereafter, to death. It is equally difficult to predict the severity and the order of the AIDS-associated conditions that will inevitably occur. Furthermore, not all patients who meet the CDC surveillance case definition for AIDS share the same prognosis. For example, an AIDS patient with Kaposi's sarcoma limited to cutaneous sites and with a CD4+ cell count greater than two hundred per microliter has a much more favorable prognosis than one with disseminated atypical mycobacterial infection, significant weight loss, and a CD4+ count less than fifty cells per microliter.

The manifestations of HIV-associated disease in adult AIDS patients take a variety of forms but can be clustered into a few common categories:

(*a*) opportunistic infections (for example, *P. carinii* pneumonia, extrapulmonary cryptococcal disease, toxoplasmosis of the brain, cytomegalovirus retinitis, disseminated *Mycobacterium avium* complex disease);
(*b*) neoplastic diseases (for example, Kaposi's sarcoma, B cell lymphoma);
(*c*) diseases of the central nervous system (for example, HIV encephalopathy; progressive multifocal leukoencephalopathy);
(*d*) non-specific constitutional diseases (for example, wasting syndrome).

Diseases in different categories may occur concurrently or sequentially. It should be noted that intravenous drug users suffer a greater incidence than persons in other risk categories of bacterial pneumonias, which are mostly caused by common pathogens of adults and, more recently, by the tubercle bacillus, as well.[11]

Wasting disease, neurologic disease, and dermatologic disorders are three of the more common conditions that produce fear and other negative responses in the patient's household. These complications distort the appearance of the patient and produce graphic and continuing testimony of the patient's physical and mental decline.

In some patients, especially those with far advanced disease, wasting can be dramatic. It is often accompanied by anorexia, protracted diarrhea, asthenia and unexplained fever. In patients who lose 10 to 20 percent of their body weight, the physical transformation is profound. The patient takes on a skeletal appearance that is initially most noticeable in the face—temporal wasting, sunken eyes, prominent cheekbones—and in the limbs. Other parts of the body are more noticeably affected later on.

AIDS encephalopathy (also AIDS dementia complex, or HIV subacute encephalitis) is the most common of the neurologic disorders associated with AIDS; it is a true slow infection of the brain. It usually develops along with other major manifestations of the disease and is a signal of profound immune deficiency. The early clinical signs are very subtle and often ascribed initially to depression or other psychiatric disorders. The patient usually complains of apathy and mental "slowing"; short-term memory is affected and reading comprehension and concentration on short-term tasks decline. Patients may begin to withdraw and to "feel depressed"; they tend to constrict their sphere of activity. As the disease progresses, both long- and short-term memory deteriorate, learning is impaired, and speech and language may be affected. Neurologic examination may reveal abnormally brisk reflexes and increased muscle tone. Profound intellectual incapacity and mutism may occur in the terminal phases of AIDS encephalopathy; many such patients also lose the ability to walk, to swallow, and to void. It is critical that important life decisions—custody planning, clarifying one's desire for various lifesaving or life-sustaining strategies, writing a will, and so on—be discussed and fully implemented while the patient is still intellectually capable.

Finally, various dermatologic stigmata of the disease can be quite disfiguring. In many patients the texture of the hair changes, becoming thin, wispy and straight; eventually some of the hair may be lost. Some patients develop seborrhea of the face, scalp, and chest, a condition that is characterized by reddened skin and moderate to marked flaking of the skin. Still others, especially gay men, may develop Kaposi's sarcoma, whose dramatic purplish-red bulging and spreading lesions can greatly alter and distort the patient's appearance.

Changing Patterns of Disease and Survival Among HIV-Infected Adults

In recent years, Kaposi's sarcoma has been a less frequent complication of AIDS in adults, including gay men; the reasons for this change remain obscure.[12] The decline in the number of cases of *P. carinii* pneumonia is probably due to the widespread use of prophylactic antibiotic regimens. On the other hand, cases of disseminated cytomegalovirus disease (including retinitis), atypical mycobacterium infection, and lymphoma appear to have increased. These three diseases, among others, probably represent the unanticipated effects of longer survival among AIDS patients in general.

Between 1987 and 1989, the average adult patient survived for eighteen to nineteen months following the AIDS diagnosis, or approximately seven months longer than survival among patients diagnosed in the earliest years of the epidemic (1981–85). The increase probably reflects the widespread use of antiretroviral drugs, prophylactic antibiotics, and accumulated knowledge of the intricacies of treating the complications of AIDS.

What Do Uninfected Children Experience?

Social Changes

As HIV infection progresses among infected members of the family, a series of events, routines, and behaviors is set into motion over which the family may have inadequate control.[13] The exigencies of the disease require close family and friends to focus more and more attention on those who are ill, thereby inevitably sucking attention away from those who are not physically impaired. Uninfected siblings may feel isolated, neglected, or tainted, but, most often, they feel worried and sad. In some families a great effort is made to conceal the severity of disease and to create the impression that all is well. Sick children cause particular anxiety in others because children are supposed to be healthy. HIV-infected children are thus often avoided—and with them, siblings and other close family members, who suffer "courtesy stigma," stigmatization because of their close association with those who are ill.[14] Some uninfected children may cope by avoiding their sick siblings or parents; others may choose to keep a secret of the illness in the family when interacting with friends and neighbors.[15] Healthy younger children in affected families often have limits imposed on their activity and on their interactions with peers. They might hesitate, for example, to invite friends to a home that has come to look like a clinic, and where much of the activity of daily living is consumed by and refocused on those who are ill. In other instances, well children in affected families may take upon themselves parental roles, providing physical care for one or more sick parents or siblings; some may attempt to protect their relatives from ridicule and condescension.

When the condition of parents and siblings with AIDS begins to deteriorate, the frequency of visits to the health provider increases. Diagnostic workups may become complex and time-consuming. In the absence of adequate child care, younger members of the family are often taken along on these frequent forays for medical intervention, further disrupting the normal daily routines of home and school and introducing the child to a new array of strange environments and unfamiliar people.

Secrecy and Lying

Because of the social stigma associated with AIDS and the well-known consequences of discrimination against those who have the disease, families may adopt one of three tactics used to protect privacy and to avoid stigma. In some cases the uninfected siblings are not told that a family member has AIDS, and any reference to disease and its associated signs is avoided. In other instances, the uninfected siblings are told of their relative's condition but are carefully instructed not to mention the "word" and not to discuss the infection outside the home. Finally, some children are told that the parent or sibling is ill, even seriously ill, but the patient's signs and symptoms are attributed to a variety of diseases other than AIDS. (Some common, alternative, vague diagnoses include "anemia" and "cancer.")

The complex psychosocial dynamics and of maintaining lies and secrets is described in detail in Chapter 4.

"Strangers" in the Home

As a parent or sibling becomes sicker, many hours each day are focused on taking medicine, resting and napping, maintaining catheters (both urinary and central venous), caring for chronic skin diseases, and carrying on the myriad activities of daily living: preparing meals and eating, bathing, voiding, doing laundry. When the patient can no longer perform these tasks or when they become too burdensome for the patient's family, outside professionals are often called in to help, and the tasks of maintaining the patient and of providing the correct array of services are divided among them. Visiting nurses may come to evaluate the clinical condition of the patient, to take vital signs, to assist with home intravenous therapy, to monitor compliance with oral pharmaceuticals, to evaluate physical findings of particular importance, and to assess the patient's degree of mental competence and emotional stability. Home health aides help with such tasks as bathing, cooking, bed changing, and cleaning. Public health nurses may intervene if the patient contracts communicable illnesses associated with AIDS—to obtain vital information about such infectious diseases as tuberculosis or salmonella, for example, or to do contact tracing for particular sexually transmitted diseases. AIDS programs that maintain family support staff may have such individuals transport patients between home and hospital, assist with child care, help fill prescriptions, and shop. Hospital-based or state government–supported social workers may make home visits to help the patient conduct routine business or to assess the adequacy of child-rearing and child care. Some families may also use the services of case managers, physical therapists, mental health professionals, and lawyers.

Young observers may find it both disruptive and disconcerting to encounter so odd a mix of people making visits to the home, to watch them in such close contact with their siblings and parents, and to have them ask intimate questions of their family members. It is equally unnerving for these uninfected children to discover that an infected relative has been hospitalized suddenly or must make a lengthy or unscheduled visit for diagnostic or therapeutic purposes. These absences from the home—both scheduled and unscheduled—add to the burden of uncertainty and social imbalance that these children experience, especially during the later stages of the disease. This is particularly true for children who live in neighborhoods beset by random crime, violence and death—a setting in which familiar persons can suddenly disappear.

The uninfected children are also likely to encounter a wide variety of medical devices and phenomena as complications of the disease ensue. Some patients are equipped with indwelling central venous catheters to facilitate the daily or every-other-day delivery of intravenous medicines. A subcutaneous port produces a bulge in the upper chest of some of these individuals; hanging from some of these devices are plastic catheters that must be kept surgically dressed and sterile at all times. Other patients require nighttime supplementary feedings through nasogastric tubes. Some may temporarily require a urinary catheter.

The child's home may gradually be filled with other appliances that transform it into a mini-hospital or a theater of the macabre. Family members— especially those with progressive neurologic disease or profound wasting —often need canes, walkers, wheelchairs, oxygen tanks, portable commodes, and hospital beds. These devices are needed because incontinence and immobility are frequent complications of end-stage disease. Children will also see parents and siblings taking a variety of drugs throughout the day. It is not at all unusual for patients to take ten to fifteen drugs each day, including several antibiotics (both prophylactic and therapeutic), antiretrovirals, analgesics, sleep medications, antidepressants and anxiolytics, vitamins, and nutritional supplements, as well as various creams, salves, and emollients. Because some medicines are given by injection, the child will see needles and syringes in the home. These paraphernalia may cause further confusion because they are often associated with illicit drug use, which children are taught is "bad for you." After all, needle use can "give you" AIDS.

In homes affected by pediatric AIDS, lives already in various degrees of chaos are introduced to a webbed complex of medical and social interventions. The social fabric of maternal-child HIV infection often includes some or all of the following: poverty, homelessness, illicit drug use, incarceration, physical and emotional abuse, domestic violence, absentee parents, and school truancy. One of the more formidable challenges for health care and social service workers is to develop a network of strategies to provide comprehensive, timely and state-of-the-art care within this setting.

Participation in Clinical Trials

In the United States, the provision of routine care to HIV-infected individuals is closely linked to the AIDS clinical trials effort. Millions of dollars have been spent by the federal government and by private enterprise to support a complex bureaucracy whose principal role is to test a wide array of drugs for their pharmacologic and therapeutic effects and to learn more about the natural history of the disease. Personnel involved in the network of AIDS clinical trials units include physicians, nurse-clinicians, coordinators, social workers, ethicists, neuropsychologists and other medical specialists, secretarial support staff, theoretical scientists, laboratory technicians, data managers, biostatisticians, and community advisers. Thousands of infected persons are participating as experimental subjects in these trials; as part of the standard consent process, legal guardians or parents provide consent to participate on behalf of minors in their care.

The trials program has provided access to newer therapies for individuals who might not otherwise have had a chance to receive such treatments, sometimes long before these useful therapies reach the "marketplace"—though some newer therapies might be no better, might even be worse, than more established treatments or no treatment at all. One of the few promises that can be given the study subject is that the data collected (even negative results) will at least indirectly benefit future patients infected by HIV.

To encourage participation in these studies and to assure adequate compliance and follow-up, various inducements are provided, including social work services, transportation costs, help with child care, and meal vouchers. Nevertheless, there are stresses, some physical and some emotional, associated with participation in these trials. Implicit in the agreement to become an experimental subject is the understanding that knowledge regarding treatment is imprecise and incomplete and that, despite the best efforts of health care workers, the illness will probably progress. The older child who witnesses the interaction between the clinical trials staff and the relative—and who observes subsequent conversations regarding the trial at home—is aware that things will not necessarily "get fixed." Furthermore, in order to assure compliance and to deal effectively with patients' inquiries regarding the study, many protocols require frequent visits to the clinic and an armamentarium of diagnostic and evaluative procedures. For families in chaos, the discipline required to complete these tasks is often new and demanding. Uninfected juveniles in these families are often "dragged along" and are intimately engaged in these encounters, and are thus obliged to assist family members in navigating the challenges of ongoing care and to pass hours at a time in hospital waiting rooms, clinics, and laboratories. These tasks are usually undertaken at the cost of the child's own developmental needs.

Notes

1. Andiman, W. A., et al., 1990, Rate of transmission of human immunodeficiency virus type 1 infection from mother to child and short-term outcome of neonatal infection, *American Journal of Diseases of Children* 144: 758–766; Blanche, S., et al., 1989, A prospective study of infants born to women seropositive for HIV type 1, *New England Journal of Medicine* 320:

1643–1648; European Collaborative Study, 1991, Children born to women with HIV-1 infection: Natural history and risk of transmission, *Lancet* 337: 253–260.

2. Ryder, R., et al., 1989, Perinatal transmission of the human immunodeficiency virus type 1 to infants of seropositive women in Zaire, *New England Journal of Medicine* 320: 1637–1642; Halsey, N., et al., 1990, Transmission of HIV-1 infections from mothers to infants in Haiti: Impact on childhood mortality and malnutrition, *Journal of the American Medical Association* 264: 2088–2092; Hira, S., et al., 1989, Perinatal transmission of HIV-1 in Zambia, *British Medical Journal* 299: 1250–1252.

3. European Collaborative Study, see note 1 above; Ryder et al., see note 2 above; Hira et al., see note 2 above; St. Louis, M., et al., 1993, Risk factors for perinatal transmission of human immunodeficiency virus type 1: Independent effects of high maternal CD8+ lymphocytes, low CD4+ lymphocytes, and placental inflammation, *Journal of the American Medical Association* 269: 2853–2859.

4. The European Collaborative Study, 1994, Caesarean section and the risk of vertical transmission of HIV-1 infection, *Lancet* 343: 1464–1467.

5. Goedert, J., et al., 1991, High risk of HIV-1 infection for first-born twins, *Lancet* 338: 1471–1475.

6. Hira, S., et al., 1990, Apparent vertical transmission of human immunodeficiency virus type 1 by breast-feeding in Zambia, *Journal of Pediatrics* 117: 421–424; Van de Perre, P., et al., 1991, Postnatal transmission of human immunodeficiency virus type 1 from mother to infant: A prospective cohort study in Kigali, Rwanda, *New England Journal of Medicine* 325: 593–598.

7. Blanche, S., et al., 1990, Longitudinal study of 94 symptomatic infants with perinatally acquired human immunodeficiency virus infection: Evidence for a bimodal expression of clinical and biological symptoms, *American Journal of Diseases of Children* 144: 1210–1215; Duliege, A., et al., 1992, Natural history of human immunodeficiency virus type 1 infection in children: Prognostic value of laboratory tests on the bimodal progression of the disease, *Pediatric Infectious Disease Journal* 11: 630–635. For a general medical overview of pediatric HIV with focus on psychosocial and developmental issues for long-term survivors see S. Lewis, H. Haiken, and L. Hoyt, 1994, Living beyond the odds: A psychosocial perspective on long-term survivors of pediatric human immunodeficiency virus infection, *Journal of Developmental and Behavioral Pediatrics* 15 (3): S12–S17 (June supplement).

8. Italian Multicentre Study, 1988, Epidemiology, clinical infection and prognostic factors of paediatric HIV infection, *Lancet* 2: 1043–1045; Scott, G., et al., 1989, Survival in children with perinatally acquired human immunodeficiency virus type 1 infection, *New England Journal of Medicine* 321: 1791–1796.

9. Tovo, P., et al., 1992, Prognostic factors and survival in children with perinatal HIV infection, *Lancet* 339: 1249–1253.

10. For a review, see A. Lifson, N. Hessol, and G. Rutherford, 1992, Progression and clinical outcome of infection due to human immunodeficiency virus, *Clinical Infectious Diseases* 14: 966–972.

11. Selwyn, P., et al., 1992, Clinical manifestations and predictors of disease progression in drug users with human immunodeficiency virus infection, *New England Journal of Medicine* 327: 1697–1703.

12. Lifson et al., see note 10 above.

13. For discussions of the nature of stressors and coping strategies among these families see C. A. Mellins and A. A. Ehrhardt, 1994, Families affected by pediatric acquired immunodeficiency syndrome: Sources of stress and coping, *Journal of Developmental and Behavioral Pediatrics* 15 (3): S54–S60 (June supplement).

14. Goffman, E., 1963, *Stigma: Notes on management of spoiled identity*, Englewood Cliffs,

N.J.: Prentice-Hall; Birenbaum, A., 1970, On managing a courtesy stigma, *Journal of Health and Social Behavior* 11: 196–206.

15. Feeman, D., and J. Hagen, 1990, Effects of childhood chronic illness on families, *Social Work in Health Care* 14: 37–53; Gallo, A., et al., 1991, Stigma in childhood chronic illness: A well sibling perspective, *Pediatric Nursing* 17: 21–25.

Glossary

Asthenia. Lack or loss of bodily strength.

Atypical mycobacterium (*Mycobacterium avium* complex) **infection.** A disseminated opportunistic infection caused by a bacterium that is distantly related to the microorganism that causes tuberculosis. This infection frequently occurs in the last stages of AIDS and affects the lymphatic tissues of the body, the liver, spleen, gastrointestinal tract and bone marrow, among others.

Candida esophagitis. An often painful inflammatory disease of the esophagus caused by a common yeast (*Candida, Monilia*). This affliction often interferes with swallowing and, ultimately, nutrition.

CD4+ cell or CD4+ lymphocyte. A particular type of white blood cell, also commonly known as a T helper cell, which bears a CD4 receptor on its surface, the principal receptor to which HIV attaches.

CD4+:CD8+ ratio. The ratio between CD4+ T helper cells and CD8+ T suppressor cells. In advancing HIV infection, the ratio is always less than one.

Cryptosporidiosis. A parasitic infection of the gastrointestinal tract that leads to profound and intractable diarrhea and, as a consequence, dehydration and malnutrition.

Cytomegalovirus (CMV). A member of the herpes virus group of agents. When cytomegalovirus reactivates in the midst of the immunodeficiency of AIDS, it can cause disease of the lungs, the retina, the brain, the gastrointestinal tract and the liver. During infection CMV can be cultured from urine, blood or affected tissue. CMV is a frequent cause of blindness in AIDS patients.

Cytotoxic T cell. A class of T lymphocyte which is capable of killing a target cell; in the case of AIDS the target cell may be an HIV-infected T helper lymphocyte.

Hepatosplenomegaly. Enlargement of the liver and the spleen.

HIV encephalopathy. (Also AIDS dementia complex; HIV subacute encephalitis). A frequent accompaniment of end-stage AIDS caused by slowly progressive infection of the central nervous system with HIV itself. The disease is characterized by disordered mentation, loss of intellectual ability, emotional changes and, ultimately, loss of motor function.

Idiopathic thrombocytopenic purpura. A hematologic condition in which the platelets in the blood become coated with antibody and are subsequently destroyed. This disease occurs not infrequently in both children and adults. When the platelet count becomes too low, bleeding into the skin (purpura) and other organs may ensue.

Lymphocytic interstitial pneumonia (LIP). A common AIDS-defining condition of older pediatric patients. In LIP, the tissues between the air spaces of the lungs and the areas surrounding the bronchioles become progressively filled with aggregations of certain types of white blood cells (especially lymphocytes and plasma cells), resulting in distortion of terminal airways, chronic difficulty with oxygen exchange, and decreased exercise tolerance.

Neutralizing antibody. A class of antibody that binds to a specific region of the virus coat and thereby prevents it from attaching to and infecting a target cell.

Parotitis. Inflammation and enlargement of the parotid glands (the salivary glands that overlie the angle of the jaw).

Pneumocystis carinii pneumonia (PCP). A severe and life-threatening infection of the lungs caused by a microorganism believed to be a protozoan parasite.

Pulmonary candidiasis. Infection of the lungs due to the yeast, *Candida*.

Wasting disease. A condition characterized by progressive weight loss that takes place over a period of months. It is not uncommon for some patients to lose 20 to 30 percent of their normal body weight. In Africa, this condition is called "slim."

Chapter 3

The Special Case of the Uninfected Child in the HIV-Affected Family

Normal Developmental Tasks and the Child's Concerns About Illness and Death

MELVIN LEWIS

Uninfected children in HIV-affected families may be exposed to a series of associated major psychological risk factors — stigma, secrecy, exposure to acute and chronic illness, death of parents and/or siblings, separations, losses, orphanhood, and foster home placements — all of which are often experienced in an environment of poverty, drugs, alcohol, violence, abuse, and prostitution.

How do the well children react to these stresses? While each risk factor has been described, surprisingly little controlled research has been published on what specific effects such stresses might have on the child.[1] At the same time, clinicians who work with such children have accumulated a rich body of clinical experience, which can provide a useful foundation for planning careful research and providing rational programs to HIV-affected families who need mental health care.

In this chapter I will draw on this accumulated clinical experience to describe how the uninfected child might feel and behave in response to such stresses. To facilitate this description I will describe two normal sets of developmental hurdles for the child: first, the set of developmental tasks each child has to master; and second, the child's developing set of concepts and concerns about his or her body, and about illness and death. For each set of developmental hurdles I will describe typical thoughts, fantasies, and behavior during the major developmental epochs — infancy, school age, and adolescence — and then describe the possible impact of AIDS-related stresses on the uninfected child's development.

Developmental Tasks

Developmental tasks for the preschool child include the establishment of secure attachments, a sense of basic trust, and increasing feelings of self-worth and autonomy—all of which derive in part from being loved and cared for by a "good enough" parent in a safe, reliable, continuing, and predictable way.[2] The typical preschool child actively seeks relationships within and outside the family and strives toward autonomy and increasing tolerance of separation from family members. At the same time the child is internalizing the limits caretakers impose. The child also acquires language, and with it an enhanced ability to express needs and feelings.

During the years of kindergarten and first grade, the child confronts the major developmental task of dealing with often intense, ambivalent emotions about both parents. Such feelings are gradually internalized rather than acted out, and they become increasingly subject to the developing internal interplay between conscience and the urge to discharge impulses and feelings and thus increasingly come under internal control.

From age seven or eight to eleven, the child is increasingly exposed to the world outside the family and learns to interact and socialize with peers and with adults other than parents. In cognitive development the child moves from a stage of concrete operations, in which the child can think logically but is still tied to perceptions, to the beginnings of formal operations, in which the child can think abstractly and reason from hypotheses. The child is now highly responsive to academic learning.

During adolescence, the individual is confronted anew by the same development tasks, but in more complex forms that require new solutions. These developmental tasks include again separating from parents and coming to terms with the ambivalent feelings toward them; developing mature relationships (including sexual relationships) with others; remastering a changing body and impulses; and defining again an identity in the context of this enlarging experience.

The special case of AIDS. The preschool child in a family living with AIDS is often cared for in a context of parental depression, unpredictability, and erratic behavior. The parent may take refuge in isolation and secrecy, becoming excessively protective of the child. In turn, the child may have difficulties establishing relationships with peers and may lack friends.

Under these strictures, the child may only develop an insecure or anxious attachment to the caretakers and a limited sense of self-worth. The preschool child may show signs of withdrawal and apathy and may exhibit such symptoms as food refusal, temper tantrums, and, in some instances, a failure-to-thrive syndrome.

Such children ages four to six may continue to exhibit excessive dependency with clinging behavior, perhaps alternating with marked oppositional behavior. Insecure or anxious attachment may also interfere with the child's ability to form or sustain relationships with peers and adults.

By school age, a child in an HIV-affected family may also have been exposed to further stresses, including serious illnesses in the mother, prolonged separations, and death from AIDS by parents or siblings. All of these stresses may lead to further erosion of self-esteem, increased depression, and difficulties in school. Oppositional and disruptive behaviors may follow failure to resolve the mixed feelings commonly experienced at this time.

By adolescence, serious conflicts may arise in each of the major areas of developmental tasks. Ambivalent feelings toward the ill or surviving parent may be manifest in severe behavioral and psychological problems, including acts of destruction and assault and thoughts of suicide. Intense ambivalence may render the conflict of separation almost impossible to resolve, leading to such impulsive "solutions" as uncontrolled defiance and running away. The child's or adolescent's fear of the outcome for the ill family member—as well as anxiety on his or her own behalf—may lead to counterphobic risk taking that includes, in adolescents, high-risk sexual encounters and drug abuse. Identification, projection, and acting out may be prominent mechanisms of defense. In this triad of defenses the adolescent, in effect, puts himself or herself in the place of the ill or dying parent and behaves as though harming himself or herself can protect the afflicted parent from harm. Sometimes the adolescent virtually invites external controls and punishment.

The clinical nature of the present database and the lack of well-controlled, systematic scientific research should provide a cautionary note. Although one or more of these reactions have been observed clinically in uninfected children of families affected by AIDS, we cannot be certain whether the reactions are specific to the dynamics within the family affected by AIDS or whether they can arise from any given stress. It is also impossible to say how common these reactions are in the well children in AIDS families.[3]

The following case illustrates the kind of clinical experience that contributes to our database:

> A 12 ½ year old boy had to be admitted to the hospital because he appeared to be markedly oppositional and destructive, and expressed suicidal and homicidal ideation. There was no evidence of any thought disorder, or of symptoms that would satisfy criteria for a diagnosis of major depressive disorder. However, there was a history of the death of the biological mother from AIDS when the boy was an infant, the virtual disappearance of the father, and marked family dysfunction in the maternal grandparents and an aunt who had each tried to care for the boy. His younger sister unexpectedly died from AIDS in another hospital while he was hospitalized. While the boy's anger and disruptive behavior was in part derived from the direct and indirect stresses caused by the AIDS-related deaths of his mother and sister, there was also much evidence of

severe dysfunction in other family members. It was therefore difficult, if not impossible, to apportion causality for the boy's potentially dangerous symptoms, including his episodes of provocative destructive and assaultive behavior, suicidal ideation, and his strong distrust of "lying" adults.

It may well be that there are many well children in families affected by HIV who are able to endure such adversity and about whom we hear very little. We need well-designed research to establish the lines of causality for the symptoms we see—and for protective factors that might operate in the environments of the symptom-free children.

Body, Illness, and Death

The uninfected child's awareness and concerns about AIDS can be understood in part as a special manifestation of the child's continuously developing concepts and feelings about his or her body and about illness and death. This development comes about through the interaction of the child's genetic inheritance with his or her environment. The child's psychological development gives rise to an increasingly rich inner life, filled with intense emotions, fantasies, fears, and cognitive constructs.[4] The inner life of the child finds expression in dreams, play, language, and behavior, all of which constitute the raw data for our general understanding of the child and of the child's understanding of illnesses and death.

Concept of Body

The child's concept of his or her body is one of the foundations for the child's concepts of illness and death. Judging from the infant's facial expressions and vocal sounds, in the beginning the infant seems to be aware of and react to pleasurable states and feelings, as well as states of discomfort arising from hunger, thirst, wetness, pain, temperature extremes, fatigue, and illness.

The infant soon learns that his or her body has a separate existence, but does not appear initially to recognize any well-defined boundary. The infant clearly sees and touches his or her body, at first randomly and then intentionally. For example, as early as age three weeks, the infant can reliably put his or her thumb in the mouth and appears to develop a schema of *thumb*. Such schemata increase in complexity, especially during the sensorimotor stage of cognitive development. The infant also experiences a wide range of sensory stimuli, including those accompanying being fed, burped, bathed, diapered, cuddled, tickled, whirled in the air, spoken and sung to, and being confronted almost nose to nose by strange, seemingly contorted faces. By three to six months the infant can smile appreciatively when shown a moving mask consisting of forehead, eyes, and nose, indicating the infant's capacity for pattern recognition—in this case, the elements of a face. The infant also begins to discriminate between sensations that come from within and those that come from the outside ("what's me" and "what's not me"). Gradually, the infant perceives, constructs, and recognizes the mothering person's face, and the mothering person's face becomes associated with all the actions of the mother that satisfy the infant. Meanwhile the infant is also further exploring and differentiating among the parts of his or her own body. The infant takes pleasure in peek-a-boo games, which help the child begin to acquire "object permanence"—the sense of what is here, what is hidden, and what is absent. The infant begins to change from watching his or her image in a mirror as though it were some other child to recognizing his or her own image. The infant remembers this image, and, usually by eight or nine months, has at least a rudimentary sense of self. All of these developments, leading up to the child's attachment to the important figures in his or her life and to the child's achievement of a sense of self and body, flourish in the context of reliable, predictable, loving, responsive, and stimulating parenting.

By the age of two or three years, the child's image of his or her body is more defined; the typical three-year-old can name such body parts as eyes, nose, and mouth, and a four-year-old can usually draw a simple representation of the body—usually a single circle with dots for eyes and nose, a curved line for the mouth, hair (by which the child usually identifies the sex), lines representing limbs that spring from the circle, and an indeterminate number of digits at the end of each limb. The child also often seems to have the idea that the body is a kind of sac filled with fluid that sometimes oozes out. If the child grazes his or her knee, and some blood or plasma oozes out, the three-year-old child may become upset at the loss of fluid. The child at this age is often readily reassured by the application of a Band-Aid, which seems to seal the leak and hides the wound from view.

A little later the child will acquire some concept of internal organs, usually from the conversations of older persons. The internal organs are usually stereotyped, however—"hearts" that look like the representations on valentine cards, for example. At this stage, the child's drawings depict bodies with floating organs, and the child has no idea of their function or physiology. By five or six years of age the body is represented more accurately in the child's drawings, with distinct head and torso, more body parts, such as eyebrows and ears, and more detail, such as clothing.

Sometimes the child's inner mental image of his or her body is represented in his or her play, especially play that involves toys that can be filled and emptied, open and shut, fitted together and pulled apart, messed and cleaned, hoarded or discarded. Gradually, with increasing cognitive development, learning, and experience, the child's knowledge of his or her body becomes increasingly accurate, although gaps in knowledge and misconceptions may persist through adolescence and even adulthood.

The special case of AIDS. The uninfected child in a family affected by AIDS may have suffered brain damage due to the mother's use of cocaine during pregnancy.[5] Subsequent impaired mothering (because of drugs, prolonged and multiple hospitalizations, and then death from AIDS) may lead to either insecure or anxious attachments. This, in turn, can limit the child's subsequent capacity to establish gratifying relationships and a secure sense of self and body, leaving the child particularly vulnerable to new stresses. The effects of brain damage and impaired parenting, especially when combined, may give rise to symptoms found in such disruptive disorders as oppositional defiant disorder and dysthymia, necessitating psychiatric treatment for the child.[6]

Concepts of Illness

Although neonates have no concept of illness, they feel and react to painful attacks on the body—circumcision of the newborn, for example, requires anesthetization of the infant. Perhaps the earliest idea of illness in the child of two or three years is as a form of punishment ("immanent justice") that has been visited on the child for misdeeds committed or imagined, misdeeds that may also be a source of guilt. Next, the child develops a primitive concept of contagion: illness is caused by a "bug," or germ, which you "catch." As the child imagines it, the germ is caught by touching something dirty or by eating something that is "bad for you." How the germ brings about the symptoms of the illness remains a mystery to the child, who may nonetheless invent a theory. By the age of five or six the child can and will ask questions and should receive simple, straightforward, truthful answers.[7]

The special case of AIDS. If the child's questions are discouraged or not answered (as may happen in the family with AIDS), the child may fantasize "answers" that are more frightening than the real ones. When a real event (like the illness or death of a parent) mirrors such a fantasy, the child's level of anxiety may increase suddenly. The child may then exhibit symptoms of an anxiety disorder, including phobic disorders, and may in some instances display disruptive behavior.

Psychological Reactions to Acute Illness

Every child has a psychological reaction to his or her illness and to the illness of siblings. The intensity of the reaction may vary with the child's developmental level and premorbid psychological state, the seriousness of the illness, and the reactions of the family. Factors that increase the likelihood of an intense psychological reaction to illness in the uninfected child can be divided into those specific to the uninfected child, those specific to the infected family member, and those that involve the uninfected child's relationship with his or her parents. The factors specific to the uninfected child include:

- young age, especially under age four;
- premorbid psychopathology.

Risk factors specific to the infected relative include:

- severe illness;
- chronic illness and multiple hospitalizations;
- difficult, painful treatment;
- poor preparation for hospitalization or treatment.

Factors governed by the uninfected child's relationship with his or her parent or parents include:

- relationships characterized by parental neglect, abuse, ambivalence, hostility, rejection, unpredictability, or inconsistency;
- psychiatric disturbance in either parent;
- maladaptive parental reactions to illness, such as unrealistic expectations, or feelings of helplessness and pessimism.

Additional risk factors that may intensify the child's psychological reactions include exposure to:

- *illness factors* (disfigurement, loss of autonomy, and immobilization, for example);
- *parental reactions* of loss, grief, guilt, depression, anxiety, exhaustion, isolation, marital strain, financial drain, and the cloak of secrecy about the illness (often found in families with AIDS).

Manifestations in the uninfected child of normal psychological reactions to illnesses other than AIDS may also intensify because of exposure to the serious illness of the parent or sibling.[8] These reactions may include:

- *bio-psychological symptoms,* such as malaise, reduced threshold for pain, irritability, loss of appetite, and sleep disturbance;
- *increased attachment behaviors,* such as clinging and demanding behavior and intensified separation anxiety;
- *regression,* expressed as thumb sucking, return to "baby" speech, wetting or soiling;
- *passivity,* with marked feelings of helplessness and powerlessness;
- *frightening fantasies* about the illness and treatment, fear of mutilation and bodily harm, and overwhelming guilt;
- *excessive anxiety,* with intense mobilization of such psychological defense mechanisms as denial, or symptoms of phobic reactions or conversion disorder;
- *reactivation* of premorbid psychiatric symptoms.

Psychological Reactions to Chronic Illness

Most chronically ill children seem to cope adequately and do not develop mental health, social, or school adjustment problems. Certain risk factors associated with chronic illness of any kind may nevertheless adversely affect the child's and the family's coping capacities, and these factors may also affect the child who is exposed to stresses brought on by the "chronic" HIV infection and illnesses in a family member.[9]

Factors that must be considered in any assessment of psychological risk for the uninfected child include the strengths or weaknesses of the adaptive capacities of the child, including the child's temperament and cognitive-developmental stage; the adaptive capacities of the parents; the "goodness [or poorness] of fit" between the child and his parent; the positive or negative aspects of the sociocultural context of the hospitalization; and the depth and duration of discomfort and pain experienced or observed.[10] Other general psychosocial factors that may affect, but not necessarily cause, an adverse psychological outcome are: lower socioeconomic status (SES), poor diet, unhygienic living conditions, and an environment of violence.

For the infected child, chronic illness sometimes entails recurrent or chronic hospitalization. When this occurs, new stresses arise, including loss of autonomy and a sense of decreased competence, relative immobilization, impaired functioning, body intrusion, invasion of privacy, and disfigurement. Parents of an infected child are likely to experience fatigue, guilt, depression, and anxiety, as well as marital stress and economic loss. The whole family may become isolated. Infected children under the age of five years may experience difficulty in attachments as a result of recurrent hospitalization. Sometimes staff caring for the chronically ill child, particularly one who is inexorably deteriorating, may become discouraged, frustrated, and angry and displace these feelings onto the child, with undesirable effects on the child and his or her family.

The special case of AIDS. A family may become overwhelmed by the implications of AIDS, especially when it strikes a child. The family may experience hopelessness, helplessness, disorganization, and numbness. In some cases the uninfected child in such a family may react to the stress with symptoms often seen in posttraumatic stress disorder: marked feelings of insecurity and greatly intensified attachment behaviors, sleep disturbances with bad dreams, school difficulties, and withdrawal.

A child, whether HIV infected or not, who is exposed to other family members who are dying or have died of AIDS, may react to the impending or actual loss with marked protest, despair, and detachment, as well as helplessness and hopelessness. A characteristic psychological reaction in the case of

AIDS is the apparent need of each member of the family, uninfected as well as infected, to keep the illness a secret (sometimes from other family members, especially young children). Typical motives for this secrecy include: (*a*) the fear of the palpable opprobrium still felt, expressed, and acted upon by some people toward patients with AIDS; (*b*) the threat, under such opprobrium, to the patient's right to education, employment, housing, and health insurance; (*c*) the patient's own sense of self-reproach and depression, which contributes to his or her withdrawal, isolation, and silence.

Whatever the forces that may lead to the concealment of AIDS, the extraordinary lengths to which some families may go to maintain secrecy are often a burden to the children, both uninfected and infected, who usually know of the infection but are not permitted to acknowledge it. This burden on the child often gives rise to intense anxiety and anger, as well as constraint and constriction, all of which may be expressed by depression, suicidal ideation, and disruptive behaviors.

The Child's Cognitive Understanding of Death

Very young children may see, experience, and understand the death of someone they know and love as an abandonment, which, the child may reason, has come about because of his or her own misbehavior. This cognitive idea, of course, is similar to the child's initial "immanent justice" theory of illness. The experience now evokes feelings not only of guilt, however, but also of anger, sadness, and loss. These thoughts and feelings are important to the young child, who needs help in understanding that the death of the loved person is not the child's fault.

School-age children who have acquired or are acquiring the concepts of universal inevitability, finality, and irreversibility, as well as the causality of death, can mourn more successfully and can use their increased cognitive and emotional maturity to deal more effectively with the feelings of sadness, anger, and guilt that are aroused by the experience of a death in the family.[11] At the same time, the death of a loved person may exacerbate the school-age child's concerns about harm to his or her body. These concerns may continue until the normative developmental tasks of adolescence are resolved.[12]

Many other risk factors may adversely influence the psychological outcome for a child or adolescent who experiences the death of a parent or sibling:[13]

- loss to a child before age five or during early adolescence;
- loss of a mother for a girl before age eleven or loss of a father for an adolescent boy;
- premorbid psychological difficulties in the child or lack of prior knowledge about death;

• a conflictual relationship with the deceased or a poor subsequent relationship between the child and the stepparent;

• a surviving parent who is psychologically vulnerable and excessively dependent on the child, or an environment that is unstable and inconsistent;

• lack of adequate family or community support, or a surviving parent who lacks access to available supports;

• a death that was not expected or prepared for or was the result of suicide or homicide.

The special case of AIDS. Children living in families with AIDS may have special difficulty resolving developmental tasks. The well child in a family living with AIDS may suffer a high level of anxiety caused in part by the prolonged and inescapable stress, the distressing opportunistic illnesses the child may witness in the infected member, and the inevitable and sometimes grueling death the child sees or knows will come. Adolescents in particular may convert their high level of anxiety to rage at the AIDS-related death of a parent. Mourning, too, is difficult for the child or adolescent in the family affected by AIDS.

Mourning

Children and adolescents have a wide range of reactions to the illness and death—from whatever cause—of a parent or sibling. It is important to recognize this individuality, especially during the mourning process.[14]

Young children may believe that the family member didn't really die (especially if the death was sudden and in a remote hospital) and will one day come back from some faraway place, or the child may have a fantasy of being seen by or reunited with the absent parent, who the child may believe is now in heaven. Young children tend to mourn on a piecemeal basis, extended over time; thus a child will most feel the loss when a previous fun time with the parent—a birthday celebration or a vacation, for example—does not happen. This event becomes a time for more mourning ("working through"). Later, a child may pretend the dead parent is just "away" and will daydream or recall memories of past times with the parent. It is not unusual for a child to want to keep something that belonged to the now-dead parent—an article of clothing, a piece of jewelry, a pen or pencil, a book or pocket knife—as a way of holding onto the memory of the parent or a token of identification with the lost parent.

Children usually hesitate to share fantasies or memories of the dead parent with other children for fear of being teased. A child may feel embarrassed, ashamed, or uncomfortably unique, gripped by the sense that he or she alone has a dead parent. These feelings, along with such emotions as anger, anxiety, sadness, and loneliness, may also become secret. As a child becomes caught in the web of a family's secret about AIDS, he or she will avoid expressing feelings and opinions for fear of upsetting the living parent.

Children work to overcome grief, in part, by expressing to themselves or others—sometime during play—their feelings of sadness. The child may also exhibit various mechanisms of defense, however, including denial. Children who lack sufficient opportunity to share feelings, or whose opportunity is actively blocked (by the veil of secrecy in the family with AIDS, for example), may resort unconsciously—or even consciously—to behavioral manifestations of their anxiety, frustration, and anger, engaging in such disruptive behaviors as marked oppositionality, temper tantrums, antisocial conduct, and high-risk behavior.

The child or adolescent must endure the grief reactions of the surviving parent, including withdrawal, avoidance, denial, and anger. Roles in the family may change. The child may become the substitute for the lost parent and take on some parental or even marital roles, perhaps caring for siblings or comforting the surviving parent. The child may feel a sense of urgency and desperation, as well as guilt in striving to perform the parental role while still in need of parenting for himself or herself.

Children and adolescents must also deal with the many changes that may occur in the family, including new partners for the surviving parent, sometimes through remarriage. The surviving parent may have to change jobs or locations, and the family's standard of living may go down.

The child or adolescent may become fearful that the surviving parent may die. A child who fears being left alone may react by becoming oversolicitous of the surviving parent, by being angry, or by acting out anxieties and guilt about the safety of the surviving parent by courting precarious or dangerous situations. Such displacement of fears, anxieties, and guilt at the same time gives the child a transient feeling of being in control instead of suffering passively the anxiety of an anticipated and dreaded abandonment.

In short, children and adolescents react to the death of a parent in a variety of ways; some cry a lot, some deny, some try to avoid thinking about it in the hope of continuing with their lives, some clamor for attention by their behavior. These and other reactions may be determined in part by the previous relationship with the now-dead parent, the relationship with surviving family members, and the inner life and temperament of the child. In any event, the young person's unique way of reacting to the death of a parent should be respected and understood by those trying to help the child or adolescent deal with his or her feelings.[15]

The special case of AIDS. Children and adolescents who lose a parent through AIDS have similar reactions to those whose parents die from other causes, but if the AIDS was kept secret in the family, the child may have a great deal of difficulty talking about his or her feelings about the death of the parent. The need to maintain the family secret may inhibit the child from expressing feelings or sharing other thoughts and fantasies. A therapist working with such a child may need to adjust the timing and depth of certain kinds of therapeutic interpretation or clarifications needed to help the child continue the work of mourning.

Mourning is often complicated for children or adolescents in an AIDS-affected family by such factors as drugs, neglect, and abuse. One pair of stresses that complicates the mourning process in these children is loss of the mother and orphanhood. By 1995 an estimated eighty-two thousand children, adolescents, and young adults in the United States will become motherless and, essentially, orphans. Loss of the mother—who was often the single parent caring for the child or the parent to whom the child was more intensely attached—makes mourning much more difficult. Shame, isolation, secrecy, economic deprivation, and cultural factors often stand as barriers to needed mental health services. More research is needed both to define the kinds of help needed and to find ways of providing that help.

Clinicians who offer group psychotherapy to both infected and uninfected children in families living with AIDS report an extraordinarily high level of anxiety in the group.[16] In the case of children who have already lost a parent because of AIDS there is an intense fear of being left alone. The anxiety often seems to derive in part from intensive dread of the anticipated death of the only parent the child has. The children in the group initially manifest anxiety by a steadfast avoidance of any mention at all of the topic of AIDS, even though they know that is why they are in the group. Only slowly and with a great deal of support do they begin to reveal their dread and anxiety. The anxiety is fueled by the embargo of the secret, but even when relieved of this burden, the anxiety remains at a high level, in part because of the reality of the actual deaths the children have seen or heard about. After the death of a parent, some lowering of the anxiety may in fact take place, as though the actual event is more bearable than the anticipatory fear. Research is needed to formulate the optimum therapeutic approach for these children.[17]

Children's Knowledge of AIDS

When do children learn about the illness called AIDS? At least two-thirds of children in first grade and 90 percent of third-graders have heard of AIDS. Common sources of information are television, parents, teachers, and friends. Thus children of HIV-affected families will have heard about AIDS even when there is a secret about who in the family has the disease. Children who have seen members of the family suffer or die from AIDS will have intimate knowledge of its ravages, of the psychological reactions of the patient, and of the ways that others respond to the disease and its sufferer.

What do children first know about AIDS? Most children learn that it is serious and probably know that it can be fatal. School-age children know, too, that AIDS has some relationship to sex, but may have confused ideas—that it is caused by kissing, for example, or even by holding hands. Children may also know that AIDS has some relation to "drugs" but again may be confused, associating AIDS with smoking or drinking.

Confusing notions about AIDS are common in children. Because AIDS is regarded as very bad, a child may associate it with cancer. Because it can be caught by using or handling "dirty" needles, the child may think contact with dirt is dangerous. Knowing that AIDS is associated with drug use, the child may believe that such drugs as cocaine cause the disease. The child reasons concretely and does not realize that it is not the drug substance but rather the infected needle and the injection route of drugs that expedite the transmission of HIV.

Given these and other widespread confusions about AIDS among children, it is imperative that accurate information about AIDS and its prevention is provided to children in pedagogically sound ways, consistent with the child's cognitive stage of development and emotional state—with a recognition, that is, of the child's understanding of illness and death and his or her feelings of anxiety, anger, and depression.

Notes

1. For a general review of the effects of HIV disease on siblings of infected children and recommendations for further research see J. Fanos and L. Wiener, 1994, Tomorrow's survivors: Siblings of human immunodeficiency virus-infected children, *Journal of Developmental and Behavioral Pediatrics* 15 (3): S43–S46 (June supplement). See also K. Siegel and E. Gorey, 1994, Childhood bereavement due to parental death from acquired immunodeficiency syndrome, *Journal of Developmental and Behavioral Pediatrics* 15 (3): S66–S71 (June supplement), for discussion of factors complicating a child's mourning of an AIDS-related parental death.

2. For a discussion of "good enough" mothering, see D. W. Winnicott, 1965, The maturational processes and the facilitating environment, in *Boundary and space: An introduction to the work of D. W. Winnicott*, ed. M. Davis and D. Wallbridge, London: Hogarth; Toronto: Clarke, Irwin.

3. See C. A. Mellins and A. A. Ehrhardt, 1994, Families affected by pediatric acquired immunodeficiency syndrome: Sources of stress and coping, *Journal of Developmental and Behavioral Pediatrics* 15 (3): S54–S60 (June supplement). Havens, J. A., A. H. Whitaker, and J. F. Feldman, 1994, Psychiatric morbidity in school-age children with congenital human immunodeficiency virus infection: A pilot study, *Journal of Developmental and Behavioral Pediatrics* 15 (3): S18–S25 (June supplement), discusses multiplicity of confounding variables.

4. Lewis, M., and F. Volkmar, 1990, *Clinical aspects of child and adolescent development*, 3d ed., Philadelphia: Lea & Febiger.

5. Mayes, L. C., Neurobiology of prenatal cocaine exposure: Effect on developing monoaminergic systems, *Infant Mental Health* (in press); Mayes, L. C., and M. H. Bornstein,

Developmental dilemmas for cocaine abusing parents and their children, in *Cocaine mothers and cocaine babies: The role of toxins in development,* ed. M. Lewis and M. Bendersky, Hillsdale, N.J.: Lawrence Erlbaum Associates (in press).

6. *Oppositional defiant disorder* is the diagnostic term used in the American Psychiatric Association's *Diagnostic and statistical manual of disorders* (1994, *DSM-IV*™, Washington, D.C.: American Psychiatric Association) to connote a child who is recurrently angry, annoying, argumentative, defiant, spiteful, vindictive, and resentful, who blames others for his misbehaviors and loses his temper. Other features of the disorder include provocative, negativistic, disobedient, and hostile behavior. Although each behavior may be present in any child, the disorder is diagnosed when four or more of the recurrent behaviors are more frequent than normal for the child's age and result in impaired social and educational functioning.

Dysthymia is a psychiatric diagnosis the essential feature of which is a chronic disturbance that involves depressed mood (or possibly an irritable mood in children or adolescents) for most of the day, more days than not, for at least two years (or one year for children and adolescents). There may be such associated symptoms as poor appetite or overeating, insomnia or hypersomnia, low energy or fatigue, low self esteem, poor concentration, difficulty making decisions, and feelings of hopelessness.

7. Children are not alone in attaching an external meaning to illness. Adults, too, may view illness as a punishment or an enemy—or as an incentive to a lifestyle change. Some adults may think of illness as a sign of weakness; some feel a sense of irreparable loss, especially following an injury. Any of these attitudes may be transmitted to the child. Upon first learning of HIV seropositivity, an adult may experience an acute identity crisis accompanied by anxiety, depression, withdrawal, and, in some cases, sexual acting out.

8. On normal manifestations see M. Lewis, 1994, The consultation process in child and adolescent psychiatric consultation-liaison in pediatrics, in *Child and adolescent psychiatric clinics of North America,* vol. 3 (3), guest ed. M. Lewis and R. King, Philadelphia: W. B. Saunders.

9. Lewis, M., 1994, Chronic illness as a psychological risk factor in children. In *Individual differences as risk factors for the mental health of children,* ed. W. Carey and S. McDevitt, 103–112, New York: Brunner/Mazel. See also F. Cohen, 1994, Research on families and pediatric human immunodeficiency virus disease: A review and needed directions, *Journal of Developmental and Behavioral Pediatrics* 15 (3): S34–S42 (June supplement).

10. For a description of "goodness of fit" see S. Chess and A. Thomas, eds., 1986, *Temperament in Clinical Factors,* New York: Guilford, 120–121.

11. Lewis, M., and D. Schonfeld, 1994, The role of child and adolescent psychiatric consultation and liaison in assisting children and their families in dealing with death. In *Child and adolescent psychiatric clinics of North America,* see note 8 above.

12. Lewis, M., and F. Volkmar, 1990, Adolescence, in *Clinical aspects of child and adolescent development,* see note 4 above, 216–252.

13. Osterweis, M., F. Solomon, and M. Green, eds., 1984, *Bereavement: Reactions, consequences and care.* Washington, D.C.: National Academy Press.

14. Furman, E., 1974, *A child's parent dies: Studies in childhood bereavement,* New Haven: Yale University Press; Krementz, J., 1981, *How it feels when a parent dies,* New York: Knopf.

15. Lewis, M., D. O. Lewis, and D. Schonfeld, 1991, Dying and death in childhood and adolescence. In *Child and adolescent psychiatry: A comprehensive textbook,* ed. M. Lewis, 1055–1059, Baltimore: Williams and Wilkins; Lewis and Schonfeld, see note 11 above; Schonfeld, D., and M. Lewis, 1994, The dying child, in *Behavioral and developmental pediatrics: A handbook for primary care,* ed. S. Parker and B. Zuckerman. Boston: Little Brown.

16. Moss, N., K. Gressens, D. Dodge, and A. Adelman, 1994, personal communications.

17. Ibid.

Mommy and Me

ADALINE DEMARRAIS

The artwork of children, coupled with direct observation and supporting information, can provide important insights into their developmental status, cognitive growth, and emotional functioning.[1] Art also functions as an expressive and therapeutic tool for children. Explaining the rationale for using art with children affected by HIV disease, Lori Wiener et al. write: "Art is another vehicle for expression of feelings and a way to reveal inner thoughts, fears, and turmoil. Children experience a sense of mastery when they complete drawings, and their finished works, especially when accompanied by a story, also help bolster self-esteem and self-efficacy. Drawings are a symbolic portrayal of the children's feelings, perceptions, and reactions to their situation."[2]

The eight drawings presented here were made by members of a support group for children affected by HIV disease in which artwork provided both information for clinical staff and a therapeutic outlet for the children. The primary adult caretaker of each of the young artists whose work is collected here was—or had been—a mother infected with HIV. The fathers of many of these children had already died (often of AIDS) or were otherwise absent from their lives. The children were asked to draw a picture of "Mommy and me" and were encouraged to include as much detail in their pictures as they desired. Children whose art is included ranged in age from five to thirteen years. All had been told that their mothers had HIV disease or AIDS.

Although analyzing children's drawings is a complicated and often quite subjective matter, certain generally accepted developmental milestones, as well as characteristic, repeated imagery, can help guide interpretation.[3] In Chapter 3 Dr. Lewis describes some of the characteristics of drawings produced by children of various ages, noting how depictions of the human body

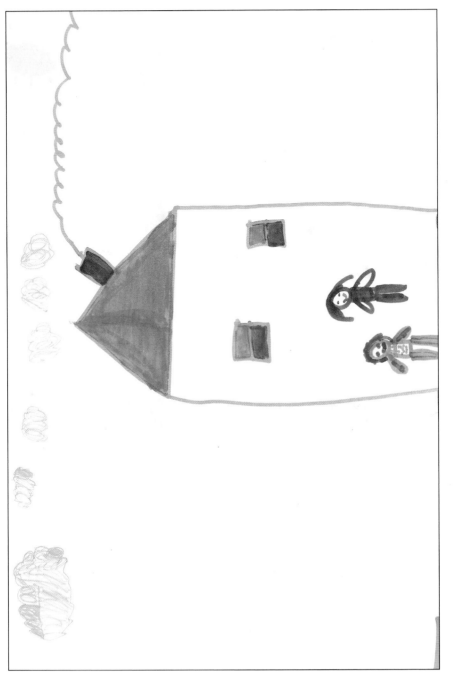

Grandma Says My Mommy Went to Heaven, But I Miss Her a Lot

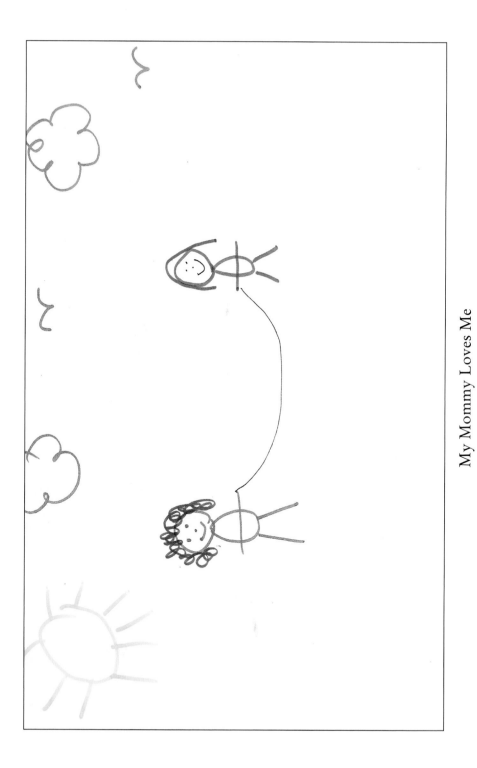

My Mommy Loves Me

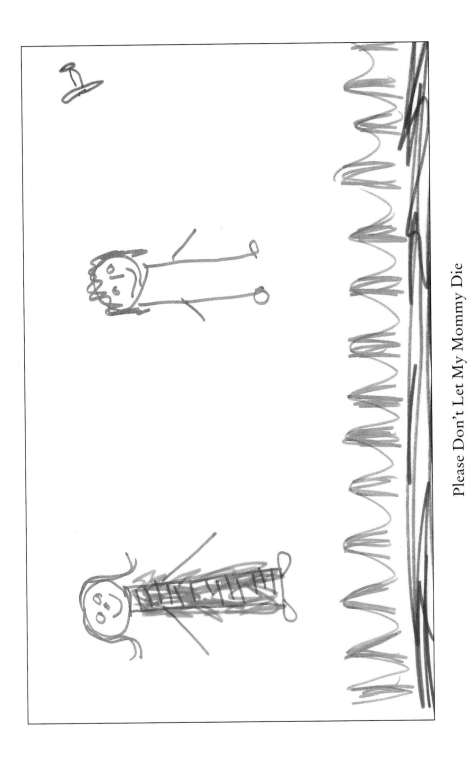

Please Don't Let My Mommy Die

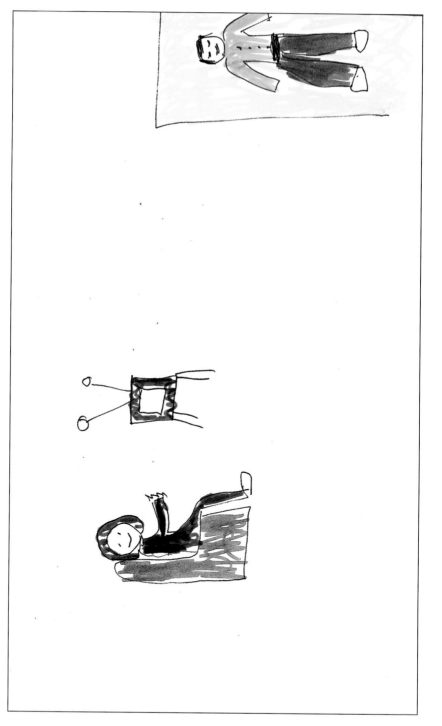

My Mommy Makes Good Cookies

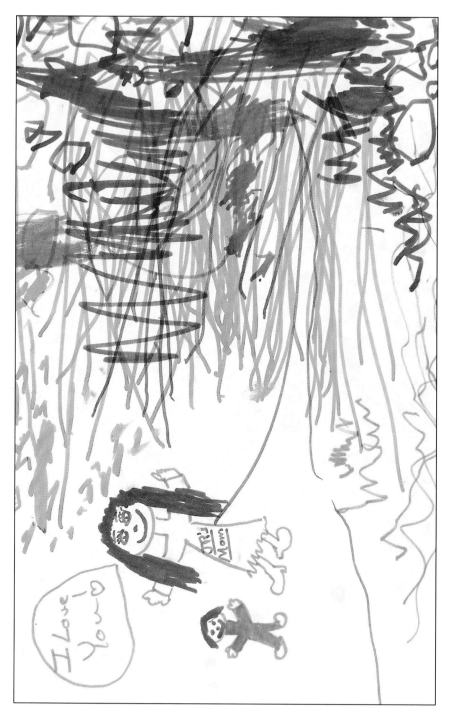

Sometimes My Ma Cries A Lot 'Cause She Has AIDS

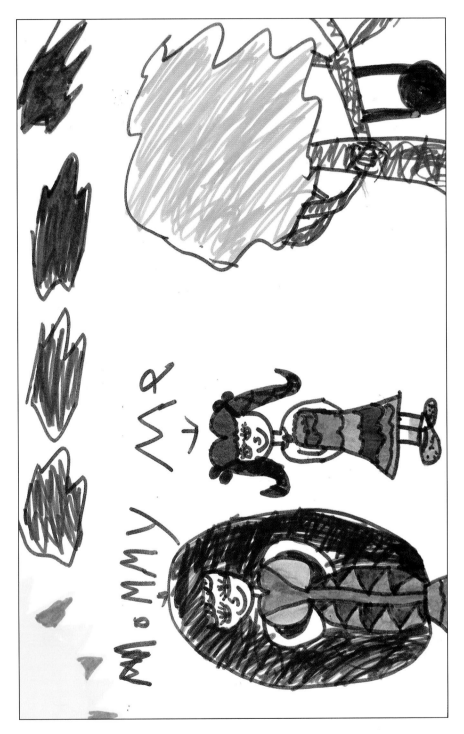

I Hate Drugs Because That's How My Ma Got AIDS

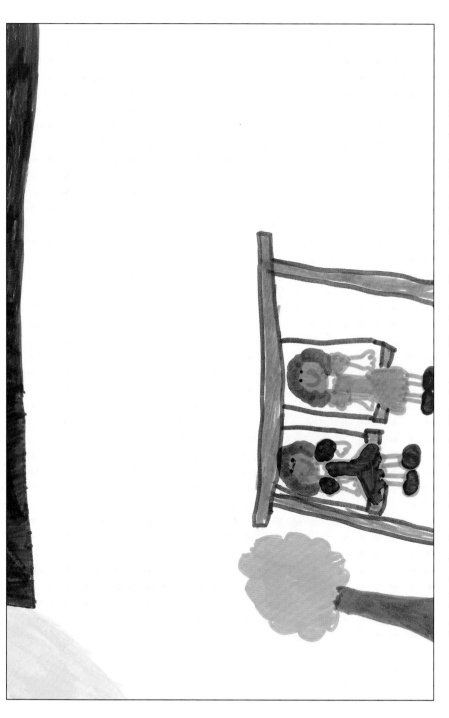

My Ma is the Best Mom in the World and I'm Not Gonna Let Her Die of AIDS

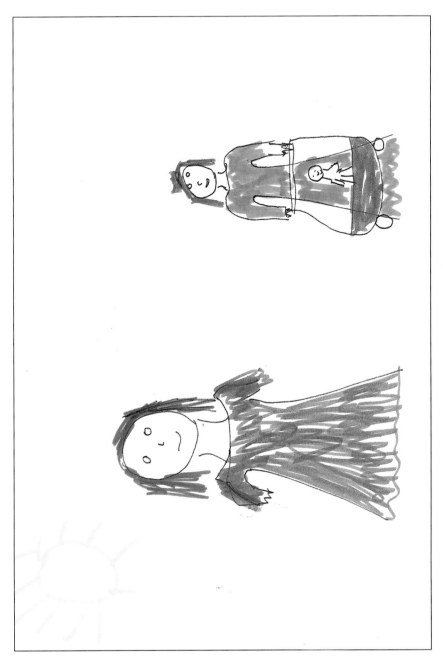

I'm Real Good Because My Mamma is Sick and Might Die

typically increase in accuracy, complexity, and detail with increasing age of the child-artist. Measured against these developmental norms, several of the following drawings by children eight to twelve years of age appear to be the work of much younger children. Many of the human figures lack hands, and most appear to be "floating" above the ground (often with no feet). This imagery can be indicative of trauma and is common among children who are feeling overwhelmed. By depicting themselves without feet, the children reveal a sense of lacking a solid foundation, of being adrift and unable to stand and face life's challenges. These floating figures may also capture fantasies of the artists—in whose young lives death is ever present—about death and going to heaven. Figures without hands commonly indicate feelings of helplessness. These eight drawings also convey a sense of isolation. Some are striking in the degree to which the figures are spatially distant one from the other. In others, where the figures are in closer proximity, children use color, form, and images to convey their sense of separation. Curiously, most figures have stereotypic smiles, and many have some representation of a sun in the sky overhead.

Each picture is presented exactly as it was drawn. The title given to each drawing reflects the child's verbal description. To assist the reader's understanding, we provide the following brief narratives, which give contextual information about each child's experience with HIV disease in his or her family and highlight certain aspects of the pictures that have special significance.[4]

Grandma Says My Mommy Went to Heaven, But I Miss Her a Lot

This was drawn by an eight-year-old girl whose mother had been dead for more than a year. The child was having difficulty accepting this death. Although the drawing is fairly well organized, indicating that she received reasonable care as a child, she now portrays herself quite primitively for her age: as a floating figure with no hands or feet, in her house which has a tiny door. The inside of the house is empty, save for the depiction of her mother, who, while better developed and grounded, also lacks hands. Her picture suggests a continuing emotional connection to her deceased mother rather than to an outside world, and her ambivalence about letting the outside world in.

A post-drawing note: This little girl is living with a very elderly grandmother and continues to show unresolved grief.

My Mommy Loves Me

The mother of this eight-year-old girl is HIV infected, but was not yet ill when the drawing was completed. Infected through transfusions, the mother seemed to feel less shame about her disease than the other mothers and has been very open with her daughter about it. Although the daughter was doing well in school at the time of the drawing, she was acutely aware of her tenuous hold on her mother. Several elements of this drawing are striking. The figures resemble those drawn by a much younger child: no hands or feet, only dots for eyes. The immaturity of the girl's figure drawing is especially significant in the face of her satisfactory school progress, which indicates no cognitive or development delays. A very thin line connects the child and mother, who are placed spatially apart on the page. This connection seems to represent the fragility of the lifeline between the child and her mother and may also suggest the child's concern that she may receive the illness from the mother or that she may somehow be responsible for her mother's transfusion-borne illness. As in other pictures in this section, the figures drawn for both mother and child are adrift on the page, floating in a sky with sun and birds, not grounded in any way.

A post-drawing note: Since completion of this drawing, the mother has died. The mother's family had been extremely upset over the illness, and alternate caregivers, outside of the extended family, had to care for the child during the mother's hospitalizations. The child's schoolwork is in decline.

Please Don't Let My Mommy Die

This drawing was done by an eight-year-old boy whose parents both have HIV disease. His father, absent from the family while incarcerated, has a history of drug use. The boy's schoolwork is well below his ability level. The drawing depicts the child's sense of vulnerability. He and his mother are floating well above the ground, each in a separate half of the picture, with no connection between them (although his smiling mother seems to be watching him out of the corner of her eyes). His mother is poorly represented. She lacks hands but has a torso of sorts, colored red (a common choice of children who depict parents who are ill with AIDS).[5] This child seems to see himself as almost nothing compared with his mother. His self-portrait is quite primitive for his age, with no body or hands. There is no sun in the picture. Rather, the boy has drawn a small airplane without a propeller (somewhat resembling a syringe), which he explained was "diving at him." The picture gives no suggestion that he and his mother are taking any evasive action or counterattacking, conveying graphically his sense of vulnerability to the threat that confronts him and his mother.

A post-drawing note: The child's father has become very ill. The child continues to perform below his ability in school.

My Mommy Makes Good Cookies

This twelve-year-old boy knew at the time of the drawing that both parents were infected with HIV; his mother was quite ill. The boy expressed feelings of responsibility for his mother and had assumed a significant role in her care. He was also beginning to experience the inner turmoil of adolescence. This drawing captures his sense of isolation. His mother is depicted sitting on a chair, floating, her body facing a blank television screen but her head turned away from it. He has drawn himself resting on a flat surface, separate from his mother and almost out of the picture. While his drawing is generally more age appropriate than others in this series (good proportions, for example, more detail in the clothing, a more elaborate face), he, too, has drawn himself without hands, portraying his sense of helplessness.

A post-drawing note: The father of this child is dying of AIDS in prison.

Sometimes My Ma Cries A Lot 'Cause She Has AIDS

This picture was drawn by a five-and-one-half-year-old boy whose father had already died of AIDS and whose mother was also ill and much less available to him than he desired. He knew that both parents had the disease because his mother, when angry, would swear at his father and say, "You gave me AIDS." The boy enjoyed drawing and, as young as he is, included hands and feet on the figures of himself and his mother, and even eyelashes on his mother's picture. In creating this picture, he started by drawing the figures, then became very angry and used the markers to create a mass of heavy, slashed, vertical and horizontal lines to which he connected his mother by a single blue line. When he grew frustrated in his attempts to print the letters for "love" in the upper right corner, he demanded that an adult help him by identifying the female figure as "JR's mother" and by writing the words "I love you" coming from her to him (which he wants to hear and to feel). His quite sophisticated figures give evidence of ability and positive development in his early years, while his slashing lines, drawn in anger, reflect the turmoil and death with which he now lives, to which his mother is linked, and which threaten to crowd in on their floating bodies.

A post-drawing note: This child has entered school and acts out his rage through his behavior, hitting other children and growing extremely angry when they approach him or his possessions. In addition, although he had been fully toilet trained, he is now enuretic and periodically encopretic, even in the classroom.

I Hate Drugs Because That's How My Ma Got AIDS

This drawing was by a ten-year-old girl who knew that her mother has AIDS and whose late father had sexually abused her. At the time of the drawing, this child was extremely angry about the impending loss of her mother to AIDS. She has drawn both figures in considerable detail and color, and like the art of other children who have suffered sexual abuse, her depictions of herself and her mother are quite sexually explicit. She portrays herself as a child who has left childhood behind. There is a strong likeness between the girl and her mother, with whom she seems to identify strongly. Both have their arms behind their backs. Her mother is drawn in a black, coffinlike object. Strikingly, with the exception of the sun, all of the objects in this lively and vivid drawing are outlined in black, and an empty black swing hangs ominously from the limb of a tree. The picture captures both the girl's clear strengths and fighting spirit (seen in her bright colors, the full images), and also her vulnerabilities (seen in the black outlines which surround her images).

A post-drawing note: This child's developing ability to express some of her anger constructively seems to have been helpful to her, for although her mother's health is now failing, this girl is doing well in school.

My Ma is the Best Mom in the World and I'm Not Gonna Let Her Die of AIDS

The thirteen-year-old girl who drew this picture had expressed her knowledge that her mother, already very ill with AIDS, was going to die. She is the youngest child in her family, and older siblings and a grandmother have assumed parental roles during her mother's illnesses. In the drawing, she depicts herself and her mother seated close together on swings, strikingly similar in size, shape, and dress, the mother distinguished only by longer legs, which reach the ground. The well-formed and colorful figures suggest that the girl has received good care through her childhood. The day, however, is not a happy, sunny day; the tree is stunted and shriveled, the sun and sky are quite abstract for a child who can draw quite well. The frame of the swing, outlined in black, appears to push down on them both. At the time she drew this picture, though she feared her mother's death, this young adolescent conveyed a sense of greater security than did many children in the support group.

A post-drawing note: Since the drawing was completed, the child's mother has died. The girl is being cared for by her grandmother, and her extended family has been very supportive. She continues to grieve for her mother.

I'm Real Good Because My Mamma is Sick and Might Die

This final picture in the series was drawn by a nine-year-old girl who is the oldest of four children. Her father died two years earlier, and her mother was ill periodically. This child was caring for all three younger siblings, had been extremely "parentified," and had been fulfilling this role for some time when she drew the picture. She has drawn her mother as almost ghostlike and quite helpless, with empty eyes, no legs or feet, and almost invisible hands. The mother appears to float near the center of the page. The child has also depicted herself with no legs or feet and only tiny hands, but, taking the role of the mother, she holds a carriage or stroller with a baby inside. The infant sibling, for whom she was caring at the time of the drawing, also was infected with HIV. Although the girl has drawn a bow in her hair and the sun in a corner of the picture, her expression does not convey happiness, and the picture is quite bleak for a child able to draw such a complicated picture of herself.

A post-drawing note: Since this picture was drawn, the infant depicted has died of AIDS.

This group of drawings is marked by the intensity of feeling that the children have expressed in their work and by the recurrent themes of drift, isolation, and helplessness. At the same time, the sunniness and apparent cheerfulness of the drawings, with their vivid colors and "smiling" faces, is in stark contrast to the actualities of much of the children's lives. This contrast suggests that the drawings might also represent a partial denial or suppression on the part of the children of their grief, mourning, anxiety, and anger—in part, perhaps, to help maintain the "family secret," as illustrated earlier in "Me on the Outside, Me on the Inside." The school and behavior problems mentioned in a number of the narratives and post-drawing notes might then represent a later, more direct expression of those feelings.

Notes

1. Two recent works illustrate the use of art and story narrative completion as useful expressive and therapeutic tools for children affected by HIV disease, whether infected or not. Wiener, L., A. Best, and P. Pizzo, 1994, *Be a friend: Children who live with HIV speak*, Morton Grove, Ill.: Albert Whitman (a picture book); Wiener, L., A. Best, and A. Halpern, 1994, Children speaking with children and families about HIV infection, in *Pediatric AIDS: The challenges of HIV infection in infants, children, and adolescents*, 2d ed., ed. P. Pizzo and C. Wilfert, 937–962, Baltimore: Williams and Wilkins (chapter illustrated by children's art). Both of these works are based upon the art and story completion narrations of twenty-four children infected with HIV and eight uninfected children whose parents and/or siblings have HIV disease. See also the recently published book of children's drawings and writing about living with the war in Bosnia, UNICEF, 1994, *I dream of peace: Images of war by children of former Yugoslavia*, New York: HarperCollins.

2. Wiener, Best, and Halpern, see note 1 above, 938–939.

3. DiLeo, J. H., 1973, *Children's drawings as diagnostic aids,* New York: Brunner/Mazel; DiLeo, J. H., 1970, *Young children and their drawings,* New York: Brunner/Mazel; Harris, D. B., 1963, *Children's drawings as measures of intellectual maturity,* New York: Harcourt, Brace and World.

4. The descriptive narratives are largely based on our personal work with these children, including our evaluation—using standard evaluation tools such as the Child Behavior Checklist and this artwork—of each child's relationship with maternal figures. Also providing extremely helpful and consistent clinical insights about these drawings were Dr. Melvin Lewis and Dr. Nancy Moss, both of the Yale University Child Study Center and its Uninfected Children of HIV Affected Families program.

5. Moss, N., personal communication, June 1994.

Chapter 4

Uncertainty, Stigma, and Secrecy
Psychological Aspects of AIDS for Children and Adolescents

STEVEN F. NAGLER, JEAN ADNOPOZ, AND
BRIAN W. C. FORSYTH

Uncertainty

To be a child in an AIDS-affected family is to be a child of uncertainty. The only certainty is the inevitable result of the illness.

Uncertainty begins for the child born to an HIV-infected parent well before the child's own HIV status has been determined. Although only about one-quarter of children born to HIV-infected mothers are themselves infected, it may take as long as six months to determine the infant's infection status. Many women first learn that they are HIV infected during pregnancy or at childbirth. Often still reeling from this overwhelming revelation, infected parents struggle with guilt, shame, and despair about their role in the transmission of the disease. Other family members who learn of the mother's infection at this time also struggle with their reactions: pity and anger toward the mother; fear for their own health; anxiety and uncertainty about the future of the infant and other children in the family.

A. J. Solnit has written that children "represent parents' replacements and hopes for immortality. These representations reflect powerful and ambivalent feelings ranging from the most intense love for children to the most fearful resentment of them."[1] For the parents infected with HIV, this universal ambivalence is intensified. A mother may experience relief at the likelihood that the infant will not be infected, guilt over the possibility that she has infected her baby, envy that the baby may not be infected as she herself is, and despair at the helpless situation in which she finds herself. These confusing and conflicted feelings are experienced both cyclically and in succession, during the immediate postpartum period and beyond. They can confound the establishment of a secure basis of attachment to the infant while the parent frets about her own role, her own infection, and the infant's future, or lack of one. An infected father must grapple with many of the same feelings (as illustrated by the story of "Matthew" later in this volume). An uninfected father who knows of the mother's diagnosis must wonder whether the child will die prematurely; he may also have anxiety about his ability to care for his surviving children after their mother's death.

Under these stresses, parents' capacity to respond to children consistently and predictably may be compromised. Overindulgence of the infected child, motivated by guilt and/or pity, often mixes and alternates with attempts at distancing and disengagement from the child as a defense against thinking about the perceived inevitable and premature loss.

As John Bowlby and others have pointed out, the very earliest relationships between child and parent have far-reaching effects on the psychological development of the child.[2] Infants of mothers infected by HIV are born into situations that can interfere with parent-child attachment, with potentially long-term psychological consequences.

Uncertainty continues beyond the initial diagnosis for parent and/or child. Because the uneven course of HIV infection may manifest itself in periods of waxing and waning health and strength, all children living with infected parents may feel the impact of the unpredictable nature of the parent's disease. Infected and uninfected children alike encounter the parents' periodic and episodic inability to care for them due to their own illness and incapacitation. Children younger than five or six, often unable to attribute these periodic withdrawals and/or departures to the disease as an external cause, may harbor fantasies that they themselves are responsible for their parents' absences. Older children may understand that their parents are sick with AIDS, yet this knowledge is a two-edged sword: awareness of the external cause for the disruptions in care includes an awareness of the ultimate loss it portends. In addition, uninfected children may feel ignored in favor of an infected sibling and may experience envy, anger, guilt, and a heightened anxiety about their own position in the family.

This framework of uncertainty, of parent toward child and of child toward parent, is the antithesis of what Bowlby has described as a central feature of the child's development of a healthy and functional personality: "the provision of a secure base from which a child or adolescent can make sorties into the outside world knowing for sure that he will be welcomed when he gets there, nourished physically and emotionally, comforted if distressed, reassured if frightened."[3]

The struggle to provide sustained, supportive relationships for their children is not unique to families with HIV disease. The effects of psychosocial deprivation, economic insufficiency, unemployment, parental drug abuse, and psychiatric impairment, as well as other chronic and fatal diseases, can all impinge upon these capacities. In AIDS-affected families, however, the issues are all the more powerful and problematic because they are compounded by the secrecy, stigma, and certain fatality that are part of living with HIV infection.

Stigma

Transmission of HIV in this country is causally associated in the public mind with both homosexuality and intravenous drug use. The linkage of a deadly incurable disease with behaviors that society has marginalized and rejected has created a social climate of fear and loathing in which some victims of the epidemic continue to be shunned and even assaulted—verbally, physically, and economically. At the same time that we repudiate these uninformed and destructive responses, we can recognize them as all too human and all too predictable.

In deep and unconscious ways, many persons affected by HIV have taken this stigma as part of their own sense of identity. On a more conscious level, children and families affected by AIDS often have what they perceive to be a legitimate fear of ostracism by the community and by their own families. In the current social environment, no one can convincingly tell them otherwise. Individuals and families thus often keep the HIV diagnosis a secret from outsiders, from immediate and extended family members, and from their own children, even those who are infected and symptomatic themselves.

Among the more commonly articulated fears expressed by parents living with HIV disease are that: (a) friends and neighbors will draw away from them if they reveal that they are infected; (b) their children will be taunted by the other children in the neighborhood; (c) their children will be taken from them by child welfare authorities; and (d) perhaps most poignantly and importantly, the stigma of the disease will cause their own families to reject them (the story of "Ann," later in this volume, discusses these feelings). Fear of the loss of the extended family's love and support is especially powerful for an infected parent who is worried about growing sicker and facing his or her own death. It is precisely at this juncture that the parent may most desire or need the family's care and assurances of care for the children after the parent dies.

The Yale Program for Children and Families Affected by AIDS has treated families in this circumstance since 1984. The following vignette illustrates the powerful effect of the sense of stigma and shame that often accompanies AIDS:

> In the program's first case of an HIV-infected mother and her children, a grandmother refused to care for her infected daugh-

ter's children, and the daughter refused to enter the hospital without a promise that the grandmother would watch them. The grandmother berated her daughter for "getting herself infected" and said that she wouldn't take care of the children because of the "shame." As the ambulance pulled up to the apartment to take the critically ill mother to the emergency room, the Yale Family Support Worker took the grandmother aside and promised to return to the apartment immediately after accompanying the mother to the emergency room and to help her find someone else to take care of the children. It was hoped that this strategy would allow the grandmother to acquiesce and to tell her daughter she would make sure that the children would not go into foster care. This promise freed the daughter—who had been placed in foster care herself some twenty years earlier—to lie down on the stretcher and be wheeled out of the apartment.

Subsequent clinical experience has suggested that the fear of telling one's family the secret of the HIV infection is often related to the patient's preexisting self-concept as the unwanted, unloved, or unlovable child. In practice, the ability of families to rally around the needs of infected children and grandchildren tends to be greater than many of our patients expect (as illustrated by Marva's story later in this volume, for example). Collective experience, however, is not easily transferred to individual patients. Reassurance is often hard to accept, and publicly reinforced fears of rejection and abandonment are powerful and persistent.

An additional and potent form of stigma that inhibits parents from talking about their infection with their children is the sense of shame and self-denigration about bringing harm to the children either directly (through infection) or indirectly (through "abandonment" by death).[4] These reactions may become particularly powerful in the context of common societal responses to the behaviors that may have put the parent at risk for transmission in the first place, intravenous drug use and/or sexual activity. The parent may suffer a sense of de-idealization, a loss of the belief in his or her own central importance and worth to the children. This challenge, most often to the mother's sense of herself in her role as parent, can bring about a depression of parental functioning, a form of hopelessness and helplessness in the face of overwhelming guilt and shame. After all, what can be more disheartening and debilitating to a parent than believing that her own "bad" behavior irreparably harmed her children?

Parents who experience this sense of de-idealization may attempt to compensate for their perceived failures by overprotecting the child, or they may adopt a distance and coolness toward the child as a way of reducing the intensity of their feelings. These reactions may oscillate rapidly and uncontrollably as the parent struggles with the guilt and shame. From the child's point of view, depending on age and developmental phase, the reactions may feel unpredictable and inexplicable. In an attempt to understand this alternating overprotection and rejection, some children will construe the reactions as consequences of their own behaviors or wishes.

Secrecy

Many families respond to the dilemma of the uncertain present and the all-too-certain future of HIV infection with secrecy and denial. Clinical experience strongly suggests that fewer than half of parents in HIV-affected families tell their children about the infection. In addition to fears of stigmatization, rejection, abandonment, and loss, some parents are reluctant to tell an HIV-infected child of his or her diagnosis for fear that the child will lose hope and become more despondent and more symptomatic. The physical effects of the illness, however, are undeniable. Most often, the result of these protective attempts is to render the disease unnamed, unspoken, and often unspeakable to children who then have no name for what they know is happening to their loved ones and to themselves.

There is a large literature on children's responses to family secrets.[5] As we learn more, however, about situations in which HIV-positive children, partners, mothers, fathers, brothers, and sisters do not reveal their diagnosis even to one another, we have begun to think that the issue of secrecy is often more about *naming* than it is about *telling* or *knowing*. Anne Adelman has explored the problem of acknowledging and naming traumatic experience among Holocaust survivors and their children. She points out that "the prohibition against naming perpetuates a sense of nameless dread and leaves remnants of unintegrable and unspoken knowledge. That which is both known and not-known permeates the representational world and constricts the individual's strategies of defense and adaptation."[6]

The majority of children we have seen individually, in families, and in groups have not been told of their parent's, sibling's, or, in some cases, even their own infection. But to say that they don't *know* is not correct. Worse, they know that something is terribly wrong, and that it is something for which they do not or cannot use the name. For many children AIDS is indeed the "nameless dread" that inhabits their families and their lives.

Clinical examples of the paradoxical and sometimes frankly unfathomable levels of denial around *knowing* and *naming* abound. Even since Magic Johnson and Arthur Ashe publicly discussed their infection and Johnson announced on national television that he was taking AZT, there are children who knowingly take AZT but don't *name* their illness; it is no longer possible to say that they do not *know*. Perhaps even more extraordinary are the adults who deliver and even accompany children, spouses, and partners to pediatric and adult HIV/AIDS clinics, and who do not *name* the illness which brings them there.

Reflecting on his father's death, James Agee wrote, "That's what they're for, epitaphs. . . . So you can feel you've got some control over the death, you own it, you choose a name for it. The same with wanting to know all you can about how it happened."[7]

Without a name, children cannot use language to mediate their experience. As they struggle to understand and cope with frightening fantasies and painful realities, they cannot manipulate words as symbols to put their fears outside of themselves. With a name they know but do not have permission to use, children are put in the position of feeling that they are defying and being disloyal to their parents every time they have a clear thought about the disease and their situation.

This pattern of conscious and unconscious concealment can have some very practical negative effects. Secrecy can interfere with medical care if patients try to avoid being seen and "found out" at the HIV clinic. It can likewise interfere with mental health care because some patients who are willing to receive medical care for their HIV infection are reluctant to accept referrals to other health care providers. In some cases, patients have accepted mental health referrals and have been in treatment for months without revealing their HIV diagnosis to their therapists.

Health and mental health providers usually strive to eliminate secrecy, especially within families. In the case of children, cognitive and emotional developmental levels are crucial considerations in deciding what is appropriate and useful for them to be told about illness.[8] John Schowalter warns about making hard and fast assumptions about who should be told, and when:

> The more painful a decision is, the more we wish to establish a rule to cover it: it would be much easier if there were an age, type of diagnosis, family circumstance, or other indicator that could be relied on to determine correctly what to tell the child. The only true indicator, however, is the child, and the only measurement is the caregiver's sensitivity. Grief is not only painful for the sufferer but also for the observer, and this is one reason why we tend to believe children know less and feel less than they do. It is not unusual, for example, for dying children to tell caregivers that they are dying, but add that others should not be told, because the patient knows that he or she is not supposed to know.[9]

From a positive and practical perspective, acknowledging the difference between *knowing* and *naming* allows care providers to work in less direct and confrontational ways with parents and children than does focusing on "disclosure." Providers can assist parents to come to terms with what their children already know and help them give the children the language with which to talk about it. This approach can be useful in both individual and group settings.

In our experience, once children have the *name* they do not necessarily use it very much. Anecdotal reports of individual, family, and group interventions tend to support the notion that children and adolescents do not routinely divulge the diagnosis or blurt it out inadvertently or inadvisedly. It seems the opposite is true. Most children and adolescents do not tell their friends. For a young child, under five or six years old, the psychological process of unconscious denial in the face of the overwhelming prospect of the death of a parent is common. Having a name for the disease that threatens a parent's life and the child's own security is important when the denial is insufficient to prevent anxiety and confusion. As episodic anxiety recedes, so the name may recede from the forefront of consciousness. However, it remains available for the child and his or her caretakers when they need to locate and label distressing feelings.

Knowing the name and having permission to use it helps older children and adolescents develop an increasingly stable awareness of their parents' and their own situations. Some will tell a trusted peer or adult in an attempt to share their burden. Most, however, will hold the secret as their parents and society have taught them. This serves a protective function for the family, but it also prevents the child or adolescent from receiving clarification, validation, and support. In addition, for an adolescent who fantasizes of a parent's death as part of the developmental task of psychological separation from parents and family, the acknowledged reality of the parent's illness and mortality can add a frightening and conflictual component to usually harmless thoughts. In safe and familiar clinical situations, however, many seem able to make good use of therapeutic support groups as a means to explore these fears and feelings.

Any discussion of the psychological effects of AIDS on children must also include consideration of who will care for the surviving children of parents infected by HIV. The stigma and secrecy associated with AIDS complicate what we know about the already difficult developmental and psychological aftereffects for children who are separated and placed outside their families.[10] In many families the reluctance of parents to confront their own illness and impending death, along with their fears of negative reactions from their family and social network, can prevent open planning for the care of the children after the parents' death. Although clinicians and caseworkers are willing to help arrange for wills and other legal custody instruments, some and perhaps many families are unwilling or unable to answer the straightforward question: "Have you decided who will care for your children after you're gone?"

The lack of explicit and apparent planning can put children at risk in two important ways. First, they may be left without a permanent home and may suffer the deepening psychological trauma of multiple placements until their ultimate legal fate is settled. The second risk, more subtle than the first, is that others may mistake a parent's inability to answer direct questions for a lack of thoughtfulness, concern, and preparation. A functional plan can exist implicitly. Social service providers may fail to recognize an existing plan for which children and alternate caretakers have been prepared because the plan has not been articulated: it has not been *named*. But in many instances the unarticulated plan has been put into action. Clinical experience suggests, for example, that many children of HIV-affected families are living in more than one household simultaneously while their parents are alive but are periodically unable to care for them. Children may spend all or part of days, weeks, or months with mother and father *and* an aunt or grandmother *and* an older sibling *and* a neighbor in seemingly limitless combination and permutation. These relationships can be supported practically and psychologically once they are acknowledged.

These plans often are hidden from outside or "official" view, perhaps because the caretakers fear that the arrangements will be viewed by child welfare and other state agencies as "poor parenting," perhaps because they don't consider such informal provisions "parenting" at all. From a practical perspective, however, providing support for these unarticulated arrangements is an effective and appropriate use of available resources in the face of a demand for foster care that may have the potential to overwhelm our existing child welfare system. In many cases they represent the best and most clinically sound placement plans for children. They address children's needs for continuity and familiarity. They allow a sense of family history and a special place in the extended family network for children. They are not abrupt or discontinuous. They simply require an adjustment of our presumptions about who and what constitutes a child's intact family from the child's viewpoint, and a commitment from social service providers to form relationships with families that will allow them enough experience and time to trust us.

Mental Health Interventions

Any program or clinician attempting to serve the mental health needs of HIV-affected children and families is advised to consider while planning treatment the unique psychological and social conditions that AIDS engenders. The following composite case illustrates some of the issues described thus far, as well as some of the difficulties and differences inherent in mental health evaluation and treatment involving HIV-affected children and families:

Christopher was sixteen months old and his half-sister, Myra, was fifteen years old when they were referred to the Yale Program for Children and Families Affected by AIDS. Christopher and his mother, Elizabeth, were infected by HIV; Myra was not. When Elizabeth was too sick to care for Christopher, he was cared for by Myra in his own home and by two maternal aunts, Karen, age thirty-six, and Norma, age twenty-seven, in their homes. His aunts lived in apartments in the same project as Elizabeth. Both Christopher and Myra were referred for a mental health evaluation by a hospital AIDS care program. Myra appeared depressed and Christopher understimulated. At the time the children were referred to the program, Elizabeth had not told Myra about her infection or Christopher's.

Although the need was immediately apparent from the referral information, it took more than six months of home-based clinical casework to prepare for a developmental evaluation of Christopher and a psychological evaluation of Myra. First, Elizabeth had to be sure that the clinical team would accept her and her family. This assurance came first by way of concrete services that were provided or arranged for the family, including food, formula, diapers, clothing, and help in securing income assistance, rent support, and utility subsidies. Further reassurance came through the persistent, committed, and sympathetic efforts of the clinician and the family support worker team to establish relations with the family in the children's interest. Often a member of the clinical team would go to Elizabeth's apartment for a scheduled appointment only to be told to come back some other day. At other times, a member would knock at the door and no one would answer.

After six months of intervention, Elizabeth still had not spoken directly to Myra about her own diagnosis or about Christopher's. The clinician felt certain that Myra *knew,* and she talked with Elizabeth about this on several occasions. Elizabeth had not spoken with her sisters, either. Her sister Karen, in fact, who was also infected with HIV, had not told Elizabeth of her own status. During the first year of intervention, Elizabeth told the clinician about a dream in which Myra found out about her mother's infection only after Elizabeth's death. Following one of several hospitalizations during that year, Elizabeth informed the clinician that she wanted to tell Myra about her infection.

The next several sessions between Elizabeth and her clinician focused on preparing for the revelation. After careful planning —Elizabeth and the clinician even role-playing the scenario— the clinician arranged a time to be with Elizabeth when she told Myra. The day and time arrived. Elizabeth was home waiting when the clinician arrived, and she said she was ready to tell Myra. However, soon after Myra came home, Elizabeth became suddenly enraged and had a fierce argument with her daughter about an unrelated minor misbehavior. It was as if Elizabeth became acutely angry so that she could hurl her diagnosis at Myra in a single breath, as if that was the only way she could get it out. Myra ran out of the apartment upon hearing the diagnosis.

Following this episode and continuing through many sessions with the clinician and family support worker, Elizabeth and Myra slowly began to acknowledge their fears to each other. Elizabeth eventually permitted psychological evaluations of both Christopher and Myra. Christopher was found to be on a generally normal developmental trajectory and to be closely attached to his mother, his sister, and his aunts. He was referred to an early intervention program that provided transportation for him and his four caretakers. During the times that Elizabeth was hospitalized, he continued to be cared for by Karen on certain days and by Norma on others. Myra was often responsible for him in the afternoons, even when her mother was home and well enough to assume her role as primary parent. With Elizabeth's help, the clinical team established working relationships with the entire family in the service of supporting the continuity of Christopher's care.

Myra's psychological evaluation was begun by a psychologist in Myra's home and completed at the outpatient mental health clinic. Myra was found to be a pseudomature, moderately depressed teenager who felt overwhelmed with her current child care responsibilities for Christopher and her anxiety regarding her mother's eventual death. Following the evaluation, she accepted the idea of a referral for individual psychotherapy. She asked that her therapist be the same clinical caseworker who had been working with the family for almost a year and that treatment occur in the home, in part because she was unsure of her aunts' availability and reluctant to leave her brother. Following the start of treatment, Myra began attending school regularly for the first time in two years. In addition to her home-based individual treatment, she began attending a support group for uninfected teenagers in AIDS-affected families, also provided by the Yale Program.

The complex effects of secrecy and stigma are evident in this vignette as Elizabeth struggles with her decision to tell Myra about the infection. Despite careful preparation Elizabeth eventually blurts out the information, as if anger was the final propellant needed to allow her to name her disease to her daughter.

This level of reticence and mistrust illustrates the importance of persistence, patience, and timing on the part of the clinician. This vignette also demonstrates the need to assess the multiple attachments for the children in the family.

That the initial referral for treatment in this case was made by the hospital

AIDS program reflects an important principle: often, the only people permitted to know the "secret" of the infection are the medical and social work staff of the HIV clinics from whom families receive medical treatment. It is frequently within the context of a medical visit that parents feel "understood" and are able to trust sufficiently to express details of their sadness, the circumstances of their lives, their concerns about their children, or the anxiety that surrounds them and impedes their need to plan for their futures.

Although the HIV clinic visit may be used spontaneously by affected families as a mental health resource, the demand for acute medical care may be so great that the medical staff lacks the time or energy for an effective therapeutic response. Despite often heroic efforts, health care providers cannot be expected to function also as mental health providers. The opportunity to build upon the relationship already established between the health care team and the family and to use it in the service of assisting family members to address psychological issues is therefore critical.

In the authors' experience, the successful provision of mental health services to children of AIDS-affected families almost always begins with the treating clinician taking the first several steps toward the patient and parent—in contrast to the more familiar mental health evaluation and treatment, in which the patient's own motivation and commitment are thought to be crucial first markers of a viable treatment relationship. The clinician's active approach demonstrates acceptance of the patient and commitment to the treatment.

A simple referral or introduction of a child and/or parent to a clinician, even by a trusted clinic social worker, nurse, or physician, is often insufficient. Patients and parents may be so fearful of rejection, or so unable to believe that anyone could make a meaningful commitment to them, that active outreach efforts and arrangements for accompanied transportation to appointments may be necessary precursors to psychotherapy. The patient may have a perceived need to assess the clinician's level of acceptance, and the time-consuming and frustrating tasks of repeated home visits and follow-up telephone calls after canceled or failed appointments may be necessary to "prove" that the clinician can be trusted and accepted.

These active first steps toward psychological evaluation and treatment present novel issues for clinicians trained to understand initial reticence and reluctance from a different perspective. The practical and psychological impact on both the client and the clinician of missed home visits and the management of the boundaries of a clinical interview in a crowded apartment are particularly important considerations in this type of therapeutic work. These and other issues require a level of clinical consultation and supervision beyond what many practitioners have come to consider routine and adequate. In addition, the impact of working with a caseload of patients, all of whom are actively involved with death and dying, must be a prominent focus of supervision and support for those who work exclusively with AIDS-affected children and families. Special attention by supervisors to the impact of feelings of frustration and helplessness on individual clinicians, as well as in-service training on issues of death and dying and peer support groups, should all be regular components of HIV/AIDS mental health programs.

Children in families affected by HIV disease are vulnerable to a host of negative experiences that may threaten their psychological growth, impede their developmental progress, and interfere with their ability to cope in all the important domains of their lives. The secrecy and sense of isolation that pervade these families also distort their relations with the outside world and challenge the ability of the mental health system to provide effective intervention and treatment.

The psychological traumas and difficulties described above are not universal. Many, perhaps most, families struggle valiantly and successfully with the myriad emotional challenges of AIDS. They nevertheless face these challenges, among others, every day. We can call upon their example of grace and courage as we attempt to meet the challenge to provide the care and support that all children and families deserve.

Notes

1. Solnit, A. J., 1976, Child-rearing and child advocacy, *Brigham Young University Law Review* 3: 723–733.

2. Bowlby, J., 1969, *Attachment and loss,* London: Hogarth.

3. Bowlby, J., 1988, *A secure base: Parent-child attachment and healthy human development,* New York: Basic.

4. For a discussion of maternal guilt see F. Cohen, 1994, Research on families and pediatric human immunodeficiency virus disease: A review and needed directions, *Journal of Developmental and Behavioral Pediatrics* 15 (3): S34–S42 (June supplement).

5. E.g., Cottle, T., 1980, *Family secrets,* New York: Addison Wesley; Roman, M., and S. Blackburn, 1979, *Family secrets: The experiences of emotional crisis,* New York: New York Times Books.

6. Adelman, A., 1993, Representation and remembrance: On retelling inherited narratives of the Holocaust, Ph.D. diss., City University of New York.

7. Agee, J., 1967, *A death in the family,* New York: McDowell.

8. Lipson, M., 1994, Disclosure of diagnosis to children with human immunodeficiency virus or acquired immunodeficiency syndrome, *Journal of Developmental and Behavioral Pediatrics* 15 (3): S61–S65 (June supplement); Fanos, J., and L. Wiener, 1994, Tomorrow's survivors: Siblings of human immunodeficiency virus-infected children, *Journal of Developmental and Behavioral Pediatrics* 15 (3): S43–S48 (June supplement).

9. Schowalter, J., 1978, The reactions of caregivers dealing with fatally ill children. In *The child and death,* ed. C. J. Schler, 123–138, St. Louis: C. V. Mosby.

10. Goldstein, J., A. Freud, and A. Solnit, 1973, *Beyond the best interests of the child,* New York: Free Press.

Chapter 5

Adolescents Living in Families with AIDS

JAN HUDIS

David is a fifteen-year-old boy whose mother, Debra, has
AIDS. His father died of AIDS about twelve months ago. David
was hospitalized following a suicide attempt shortly after his
father's death.

David lives with his mother and his twelve-year-old brother,
Michael. His seventeen-year-old sister has lived with their
maternal grandmother for the last two years. It takes David
about an hour on public transportation to travel from his home
to his grandmother's home.

Debra is overwhelmed by the changes which have taken place
in her life since her husband was diagnosed as HIV infected three
years ago. She experiences periods of deep depression and
drinks heavily. Though she belongs to an alcoholism counseling
group, she rarely attends meetings. On the surface, she may
appear to be coping with her difficulties; in reality, she is barely
holding on.

David and his siblings have expressed a great deal of anger
toward Debra. They feel she failed to adequately care for their
father when he was ill, and they blame her for his death. Their
anger is compounded by Debra's failure ever to speak with them
about the cause of their father's death or about her own illness.
They learned about their parents' diagnoses from hostile
comments made by neighbors.

Debra is unable to handle the tasks of parenting and has little
control over the behavior of her children, especially David. He
is often "out of control" and self-destructive. He is described by
his mother and the case manager working with the family as a
"nightmare" and a "terror." Occasionally he stays out all night
and threatens his mother with violence if she protests. He is
disruptive in class, has assaulted teachers, and is often truant or

suspended from school. An average student in a mainstream classroom at the time of his father's diagnosis three years ago, David has since been moved to progressively more structured special education settings. His standardized tests show no sign of developmental delay or learning disability; his placement in special education is solely attributable to his behavior. Six months ago, David was sent to live in a group home. He ran away from it and has made it clear that he will never return.[1]

No one knows how many adolescents survive AIDS in their families. But if estimates vary, all agree that the numbers are large and increasing rapidly. In New York City alone, estimates range from 6,700 adolescent survivors by the end of 1994 to 26,000 survivors in 1995.[2] The experiences of the adolescent survivors of families with AIDS—and the challenges they present—differ in significant respects from those of their younger siblings. These adolescents find themselves in situations that demand a level of maturity beyond their years and that bind them even more tightly to their families at the very time they seek the normal emancipation of adolescence. Society often fails to acknowledge their experience or support them as they struggle to cope with great loss and to learn the skills needed to be independent. Some respond well to these challenges. Others do not.

Many adolescents living in families with HIV disease are called upon to assume caretaking responsibilities for younger siblings and ill parents; some may miss many days of school while others may drop out, thereby increasing their isolation from social supports. Placement for these adolescents after their parents' deaths can be extremely difficult, especially if they have been functional heads of household, are "acting out," or want to establish a new household as guardians for their younger siblings.

The complex stressors occasioned by AIDS in the family further complicate the difficult normative demands of adolescence, a time for testing limits and developing a sense of self. These youths become particularly vulnerable during the illness and following the death of their parents. They often respond by engaging in high-risk behaviors, such as frequent unprotected sexual intercourse with multiple partners. Their unique needs are just beginning to be recognized, and far too few services exist to meet them.

This chapter reviews some of the unique challenges that AIDS poses to surviving adolescent family members, suggests ways to improve our responsiveness to their needs, and proposes a research agenda. Data on these "well" adolescents are extremely limited. In describing the problems they face, this chapter draws from two primary sources: a formal assessment of adolescent mental health needs conducted by the New York City Human Resources Administration Division of AIDS Services (DAS) in 1991 and the anecdotal reports of DAS caseworkers concerning well adolescents in families with AIDS over more than three years of intensive work with these adolescents and their families.

The Needs of Well Adolescents in Families with AIDS

Current Understanding of Adolescent Response to Family AIDS-Related Deaths

Adolescent bereavement has not been the subject of substantial scholarly research.[3] Virtually no studies have followed an adolescent cohort prospectively to study their bereavement responses.[4] Recent studies indicate that bereaved adolescents are more likely than their peers to be emotionally distressed and to experience behavior problems and impaired social relationships.[5] They may be at special risk for multiple behavior problem syndrome, which can include frequent unprotected sexual intercourse with multiple partners, problems with conduct, and substance abuse.[6] Adolescents may respond to parental deaths by withdrawing.[7] Unfortunately, no controlled, prospective research has been completed which specifically concerns the response of adolescents living in families with AIDS, though at least one such study is in progress.[8] Professionals who counsel these adolescents, however, often observe that they assume the ill parent's family responsibilities when the parent becomes ill and that they may concurrently feel neglected and envious when all adult attention in the family is diverted to sick parents and siblings.[9] These adolescents also may experience excessive separation conflicts with the parent infected by HIV, especially when the adolescent knows the parent's prognosis.[10] Support groups for these adolescents may be helpful in heightening their empathy and sensitivity, improving their school performance, and decreasing their anger, anxiety, and negative behaviors, but these groups are unavailable to adolescents whose parents keep the diagnosis a secret.[11]

Design of the Adolescent Needs Assessment

In 1991, as part of its ongoing commitment to identify client needs and to design innovative programs to address those needs, DAS conducted a cross-sectional study of the mental health needs of well adolescents in families with AIDS.[12] Using pilot funds from the National Institute of Mental Health and the federal Health Resources and Services Administration, the study used face-to-face, in-home interviews of the adolescents and their parents/guardians (averaging three hours each), genograms, and quantitative standardized instruments to assess the adolescents' self-esteem, anxiety, and depression. Fifty-nine adolescents from forty families were interviewed. (Twenty-seven percent of the families originally contacted refused to participate.) In twenty of these forty families the parent with AIDS was still alive and living in the household. In the other twenty the parent had died of AIDS in the last six months and the adolescent was living with a new guardian. The families interviewed were 42 percent African-American and 58 percent Hispanic (an ethnicity that generally reflects the DAS family caseload, except that 9 percent of DAS family cases are white). Youths interviewed ranged in age from ten years through nineteen (49 percent were ten to thirteen; 41 percent were fourteen to seventeen, and 10 percent were eighteen to nineteen). AIDS was not mentioned in the interview until—and unless—the parent, guardian, or adolescent mentioned it. Interviews were conducted with the common understanding that the purpose of the assessment was to understand the needs of well adolescents in families in which there was a serious illness.

The Experience of Well Adolescents in Families Living with AIDS

The final report of the needs assessment identifies four primary themes that characterize the experience of well adolescents in families living with AIDS: (*a*) multiple losses; (*b*) isolation and lack of social supports; (*c*) destructive coping behaviors; and (*d*) problems identifying and maintaining new custodial placements.[13]

Loss. Loss, related and unrelated to AIDS, was a predominant theme in the lives of the adolescents interviewed in the needs assessment. The mean number of major losses (through death, divorce, or incarceration of significant others, for example) experienced by the adolescents in the previous two years was four. More than 80 percent had experienced at least one such major loss. Absent fathers were common; the youths had learned to expect that their fathers would visit rarely and often would be in jail. When one youth was asked whether he ever visited his father in prison, he responded, "Why should I? I never see him when he is out." The adolescents talked about these losses with an eerie matter-of-factness. "We just have to move on" was the typical response when they were asked about the personal impact of a loss.

Isolation. These losses, and the associated changes in living situation, neighborhood of residence, and school, often result in significant isolation of these youths from their peer and adult social networks.[14] In families with limited economic and transportational resources, a move to a new neighborhood and/or school is almost always associated with significantly reduced contact and a loosening of bonds with neighborhood and school friends. Only a few youths were able to remain in their own homes, when the new guardian, usually a grandmother, moved in to care for the dying parent and then remained after the parent's death. Thirty-eight percent of the youths in the needs assessment reported that they had no best friend; four of them said that they did not have anyone they considered a friend.

The stigma surrounding AIDS further compounds the adolescents' sense of isolation. Of families interviewed in the needs assessment, very few had chosen to reveal their HIV status outside the family. Some of the parents interviewed and many of those who had died chose not to inform some or all of their children, often out of a desire not to burden them with the knowledge or a fear that the youths would inadvertently reveal the parent's HIV status to others. Only 61 percent of the youths reported that they knew the HIV status of their parent; almost all of them had been specifically instructed not to speak about it with anyone outside the family. In several cases, adolescents reported that the parent had cancer, though the study interviewers had been told that the youths knew about HIV in the family. Of those youths who both knew and who reported having a best friend, none had told the best friend. This was true even for a youth who knew her best friend's mother also had AIDS.

Many youths seemed to understand the toll that this "secret keeping" took on their access to informal and formal social support networks. One of the most touching stories the interviewers were told during the course of the needs assessment was a mother's account of the experience of her twelve-year-old son, Raphael, when a classmate revealed that her mother had AIDS. Pandemonium ensued, and all the children physically withdrew from the child. Raphael did the same, and felt terrible about doing so. He related the story to his mother because he felt that he had abandoned a classmate whose experience was so similar to his. He had feared that to be supportive in any way might have been interpreted as an admission that his family was also affected by AIDS, a risk he was not prepared to take.

Negative coping behaviors. Adolescents interviewed for the needs assessment exhibited a wide range of responses to the stress of living with a parent with AIDS. Some responses were supportive; others were self-destructive. Thirty-four percent of the parents/guardians reported that the youths were "acting out" at home and/or school (for example, truancy, disruptive behavior resulting in school suspension or arrest, defiance of parental rules, or running away without informing parents of their whereabouts for days). Twenty-five percent of the boys had recent experience with law enforcement, including three who had been incarcerated. Seventy-three percent of the youths reported problems in school, and 58 percent reported a decline in school grades associated with parental illness.[15] A number of older adolescents had been suspended from school; others dropped out (for girls, pregnancy was often the given reason). Only one of the older adolescents mentioned a school staff person who was aware of his loss and acted as an advocate—the boy's football coach, whose loss of his own mother as a teen fostered the growth of this strong connection. Little drug use was reported, but boys and girls alike reported having unprotected sex. Of the five older adolescent girls who reported having had sex, four reported being pregnant at least once. Parents reported decreasing influence over their adolescents' behavior as their illness progressed, in part because they became less able to supervise and in part because they feared that discipline would threaten their already tenuous relationship with the youths.

These data revealing significant "acting out" behavior by many of these youths have been corroborated in early analysis from a prospective NIMH-funded study of 360 adolescents in families with AIDS in New York City, which seeks to evaluate the effectiveness of interventions designed to reduce negative outcomes for these youths.[16] Baseline assessment data for the first forty-seven adolescents interviewed in this ongoing study indicate that in the last six months: (a) 72 percent reported being in a serious physical fight where there was punching or hitting; (b) 13 percent had been arrested and gone to court for illegal activity; and (c) 2 percent had gone to jail. One-third of the youths reported that they would be in more trouble if the police knew everything that they had done.

Problems identifying and maintaining custodial placements. In the needs assessment, it appeared to the interviewers that age was a key factor in a young person's adjustment to the parent's illness and death, and to the associated changes in living situation. From ages ten to twelve years, the youths were more compliant and in less conflict with parents and guardians. Arranging custody placements for older adolescents was particularly problematic; many were in such conflict with adult authority figures that they frequently moved from one living situation to another.

In the needs assessment, there was no viable custody plan for more than half the adolescents in families in which the parent was still living. David's case is illustrative of one type of difficulty. For him, there is no custody plan in place and the mother has little hope that she will be able to develop one before she dies; no one in her family will take responsibility for an abusive, "acting-out" teenager, though of all her children his future concerns her the most. She fears that his knowledge that there is no plan for his custody will further strain his ability to cope with the stress of her deteriorating health. The experience of caseworkers at DAS indicates that older youths with deteriorating home lives and no viable custody plan are often destructive to themselves or others; some make choices that limit their maturation into independent adulthood. Boys may end up in jail and girls may become pregnant (becoming eligible for public assistance independent of another adult). In either circumstance, the youth's situation tends to restrict, rather than promote, growth and development into a productive, independent adult.

Other families face different placement dilemmas. In some, the older teenager may be the only person able to assume permanent custody of the younger children when the parent dies. In others, family members may be willing to take custody of the younger siblings but not the older youth. When siblings insist upon remaining together as a family after being orphaned, older adolescents may go to great lengths to keep everyone together under one roof. In one DAS family, the oldest adolescent became embroiled in a court battle against other relatives over who would have custody of the younger children. The oldest adolescent in another family, determined to secure custody of her two younger siblings, deliberately had a baby so she could establish an independent welfare case and show that she was capable of heading a household. For adolescents accustomed to acting as "head of household" during the parent's illness, placement with a new family in which they are expected to return to a dependent role can create great conflict.

Cultural issues may also be particularly problematic if the grandmothers who seek to help have lived much of their lives outside the United States (often in rural areas) while their grandchildren grew up in United States cities. The potential for misunderstanding and conflict is great in these situations, as the youth may not speak the grandmother's native language and almost certainly has grown up with different cultural norms and expectations.

The Role of AIDS

Policymakers and researchers may properly question to what extent the experiences of adolescents described by the needs assessment are directly attributed to AIDS in the family. Is there something unique about these youths that justifies special attention and resources to meet their needs? The question is difficult to answer with current data. The rates of delinquency behavior, school suspension, unprotected sexual intercourse, teenage pregnancy, and drug and alcohol use are already high in the communities most affected by AIDS, and the few studies completed on this adolescent population (including the needs assessment discussed here) have lacked a control group of youths faced with similar stressors from poverty, substance abuse, severe family discord, and violence in their homes and communities, but free from HIV disease in their families. We know, however, that families living with AIDS experience some unique types of stress, and that uninfected family members may experience stress as great as that reported by the ill family member or members.[17] Indeed, the strain on adolescent family members may well be even greater than that experienced by younger siblings because they not only must cope with the difficult normative demands of their own adolescence but may also feel obligated to assume, concurrently, the role of parent.

Addressing the Needs of Well Adolescents in Families with AIDS

Any plan to develop specialized services for these well adolescents must confront the question of whether to address just the needs of these adolescents who have HIV disease in their families or to act more broadly to address unmet needs of all youths whose behaviors or environments suggest that they are at risk of poor outcomes in our schools, juvenile courts, and child welfare systems. Both are necessary. Programs must be developed to address the needs of all adolescents at risk, but these programs must also recognize the special service requirements of youths affected by AIDS. In addition, specialized services for youths affected by HIV must confront directly the issue of stigma. Will youths willingly use these services, or will the services themselves assume a stigma, deterring youths from seeking them? This concern is important because the services should be as accessible as possible for all youths.

The following changes would markedly improve our response to well adolescents living in families with AIDS:

• *Professional training and advocacy.* These youths need advocates in the school and court systems. Professionals who are likely to work with them (teachers, school nurses, attorneys, judges, juvenile justice personnel) need training to foster an awareness that a youth's "acting out" behavior could be in reaction to an AIDS-related illness or death. School advocacy is needed to guide a youth with family caretaking responsibilities to helpful alternative educational settings (GED programs, magnet schools) and approaches that demonstrate sensitivity to their unique needs (including a flexible school schedule). Training for judges could influence the types of treatment offered to these youths, since many may need intensive follow-up, job skills training, and bereavement counseling, especially when they are released back into the community from juvenile justice facilities. Many youths released into the community also need intensive assistance in finding housing.

• *Mental health services.* These youths and their families have significant mental health needs, yet most lack even a supportive structure for bereavement and healing. Their needs are not adequately addressed by the community mental health system for several reasons: (*a*) lack of understanding by the treating professionals of youths' unique needs; (*b*) long waiting lists; and (*c*) ethnic and language barriers. Lack of available transportation options that are acceptable to families is another major obstacle, especially for youths who seek services outside their neighborhood to maintain confidentiality. (A fourteen-year-old Bronx girl, who expressed a desire to attend a support group for youths who had recently lost parents, grew frustrated because the group, one of the few in New York City, met in Manhattan and she was too young to travel there by subway.)

• *Grief counseling.* Often, AIDS-specific group counseling for adolescents is difficult to organize and sustain.[18] One group in New York City, organized by a practitioner specializing in individual counseling for children of parents with AIDS, took three years to assemble. Mixing boys and girls in a group may prove problematic for younger adolescents, as may mixing youths from different ethnic backgrounds. Groups designed to help adolescents develop and enhance their ability to cope with a parent's chronic illness and to plan for their future are being tested in the ongoing prospective NIMH intervention study. Though we do not yet know the long-term impact of such groups on these adolescents, in the short-term participants report much peer support and sharing.

• *Enhancing the schools' role.* Schools provide an appropriate forum for generic forms of group counseling services that can help youths with all types of loss, including AIDS-related loss, so prevalent in many of these communities. At least one very successful program in New York City is being operated by a community-based agency in a school district. Students come to talk about loss, but not necessarily the reasons for those losses. Some youths eventually reveal that their losses are HIV related.

• *Viable placements.* It may be possible to increase the viability of out-of-home placements for these youths by: (*a*) recruiting foster parents specifically to provide homes for adolescents and providing them with intensive training and case management; (*b*) revisiting "traditional" residential treatment models, like residential schools, either in non-urban areas or in housing where residency is contingent upon school attendance and satisfactory performance; and (*c*) creating supported housing options (rather than just independent-living housing, which establishes youths in their own apartments but provides no ongoing supports).

• *Training for independent living.* These youths have vastly different abilities to live independently. Some need very little support before they are ready to assume full responsibility for themselves, but most youths coming from dysfunctional families have had such poor in-family, in-home training that the bridge time for them will be extremely long. They need basic instruction in such matters as structuring their time and their living arrangements, basic social skills (how to dress, how to address others), and day-to-day routines (what to expect, for example, upon going to a bank to open a bank account or ordering food at a restaurant). Fully independent housing options do not make sense for most of these youths until they have received such basic training.[19]

• *Workplace training and mentoring programs.* Jobs can be important bridges to independence. In the needs assessment, when youths were asked what they most wanted, the majority answered, "a job." Employment is difficult for these youths to secure, sometimes because jobs are not available, but more often because the youths lack the skills needed to secure even the most basic employment. Through workplace mentorship programs, youths can be introduced into work environments in a way that provides them with both group support and basic job training.

• *Community-based mentoring programs.* Mentoring programs based in the community can provide important opportunities for a youth to try new skills with guidance of an adult who can assist if a mistake is made. For many of these youths, one mistake in an unfamiliar situation can be so devastating that it becomes an obstacle to all additional attempts to master that situation. Many AIDS-affected youths need significant mentoring before they can become a part of any culture other than that of the streets.

• *Services for adolescent guardians.* Modifying the law to allow co-guardian-ship arrangements could allow an older adolescent to become the primary guardian for younger siblings yet provide an adult "proxy" guardian. This adult could provide respite guardianship, backup guardianship (if the adoles-cent proved to be no longer interested in, or capable of, being guardian), and ongoing encouragement and help with problems. Adolescent guardians also can benefit from skill-building training in parenting and in family communi-cation, with ongoing professional backup support to assist them in responding to the developmental and psychosocial needs of their siblings.

• *Health education.* The high frequency of unsafe sexual practices among these adolescents is of great concern. Youths on the DAS caseload appear more aware of the linkages between drug use behavior and AIDS than of those between unsafe sexual behavior and AIDS. We must conduct research to assess why that is, and what we can do to change it.

In addition, because data about these adolescent survivors are so sorely lacking, we must pursue a vigorous research agenda. Qualitative as well as quantitative research is necessary. Specific questions of interest include:

• How do guardianship arrangements differ in families with and without a child who is also infected with HIV?

• How can the experience of adolescents who have successfully survived tran-sition into new families be shared with others? Can an adolescent serve as a mentor to other adolescents during their transitions?

• What are the consequences of long-term co-parenting (which occurs when the sole remaining parent, who has chosen a new guardian for her child, lives longer than expected) on these adolescent survivors and their younger sib-lings? One often observes tremendous conflict over the parental role between the parent and the new guardian, putting the youth into a very difficult posi-tion.

• What are the long-term effects on adolescents of a parental death, and how might these effects differ when the death is from a stigmatizing illness like AIDS?

As the number of people with AIDS continues to climb, services for fami-lies will need to be expanded. Adolescent survivors of AIDS in their families have special needs that must be addressed if these youths are to deal con-structively with the loss and trauma of AIDS that currently devastate their families and communities. It is essential to create strategies that will ensure secure, stable living situations in which these adolescents can choose school, work, and hope over pregnancy, drugs, and violence. Failure to invest now in the research and design of programs that help adolescents and their families develop stable living situations and make productive, positive choices will only delay society's payment for services for this population.

Notes

1. David's story illustrates the fragmentation that often occurs in families with AIDS, as illness strains already-fragile coping skills of parents, children, and other family members. Family fragility is often compounded by substance abuse and poor communication, as is seen in David's family. As youths like David seek ways to cope with their own anger and the increasingly chaotic situation at home, they often display negative coping behaviors, hurting themselves and others. This behavior often results in their being placed in increasingly restrictive environments, such as juvenile detention and special education.

2. For estimate of 6,700, see C. Levine and G. Stein, 1994, *Orphans of the HIV epidemic: Unmet needs in six U.S. cities,* New York: The Orphan Project. For estimate of 26,000, see C. Norwood, 1989, AIDS orphans in New York City: Projected numbers and policy demands, *International Conference on AIDS* 5: 840; Drucker, E., et al., 1988, *IV drug users with AIDS in New York City: A study of dependent children, housing and drug addiction treatment.* Manuscript. New York: Montefiore Medical Center, Department of Epidemiology and Social Medicine.

3. Raphael, B., 1983, *The anatomy of bereavement,* New York: Basic; Dane, B., and S. Miller, 1992, *AIDS: Intervening with hidden grievers,* Westport, Conn.: Auburn House; Gersten, J., J. Beals, and C. Kallgren, 1991, Epidemiology and prevention interventions: Parental death as a case example, *American Journal of Community Psychology* 19: 481–500.

4. Weller, E., and R. Weller, 1991, Grief. In *Child and adolescent psychiatry: A comprehensive textbook,* ed. M. Lewis, Baltimore: Williams and Wilkins, 389–394; Harris, E., 1991, Adolescent bereavement following the death of a parent: An exploratory study, *Child Psychiatry and Human Development* 21 (4): 267–281.

5. For an excellent discussion of adolescent response to AIDS-related deaths in family, see chapter 4, Intervening with children and adolescents, in Dane and Miller, note 3 above. See also S. West et al., 1991, The use of structural equation modeling in generative research: Toward the design of a preventive intervention for bereaved children, *American Journal of Community Psychology* 19: 459–480.

6. Windle, M., 1991, Problem behavior in adolescence, in *Encyclopedia of adolescence,* ed. R. M. Lerner, A. C. Peterson, and J. Brooks-Gunn, 2: 839–844. New York: Garland; Ensminger, M. E., 1990, Sexual activity and problem behaviors among black, urban adolescents, *Child Development* 61: 2032–2046; Irwin, C., and S. Millstein, 1991, Risk-taking behaviors during adolescence, in *Encyclopedia of adolescence,* 2: 934–943.

7. Raphael, B., et al., 1990, The impact of parental loss on adolescents' psychosocial characteristics, *Adolescence* 25: 689–700; Osterweis, M., F. Solomon, and M. Green, 1984, *Bereavement: Reactions, consequences, and care.* Washington, D.C.: National Academy Press.

8. A June 1994 report on the published literature found no empirical studies of the grief reactions of "AIDS orphans" of any age. See K. Siegel and E. Gorey, 1994, Childhood bereavement due to parental death from acquired immunodeficiency syndrome, *Journal of Developmental and Behavioral Pediatrics* 15 (3): S66–S71 (June supplement). The study in progress is Rotheram-Borus, M. J., and B. Draimin, 1992, Interventions for adolescents whose parents live with AIDS. NIMH Grant MH49958-03.

9. Fanos, J., and L. Wiener, 1994, Tomorrow's survivors: Siblings of human immunodeficiency virus-infected children, *Journal of Developmental and Behavioral Pediatrics* 15 (3): S43–S48 (June supplement); Dane and Miller, see note 3 above; Evans, M., et al., 1994, Counselling HIV-negative children of parents with HIV disease: A structured protocol, *AIDS Patient Care,* February, 1994: 16–19; Wiener, L., and A. Septimus, 1994, Psychosocial support for child and family, in *Pediatric AIDS: The challenge of HIV infection in infants, children, and adolescents,* ed. P. A. Pizzo and C. M. Wilfert, Baltimore: Williams and Wilkins, 809–828; Nehing,

W., K. Malm, and D. Harris, 1993, Family and living issues for HIV-infected children. In *Women, children, and HIV/AIDS,* ed. F. Cohen and J. Durham, New York: Springer.

10. Evans et al., see note 9 above.

11. Wiener and Septimus, see note 9 above.

12. DAS was established in 1987 to serve the special needs of Medicaid-eligible persons with advanced HIV disease by coordinating their health care, welfare, housing, and home care services. Its Family Unit provides case management, as well as family counseling and social support services, to enable households affected by AIDS to remain together as long as possible. Since the beginning of the epidemic, DAS has managed nearly fifty thousand cases, including about eight thousand family cases. Its family caseload has grown from an average of three hundred per month in 1988 to nearly three thousand in February, 1994. Over 90 percent of these families are Latino or African-American, and the majority of the households are headed by single women, many of whom have a history of substance abuse. Of these families, about 40 percent have at least one adolescent in the household.

13. Draimin, B. H., J. Hudis, and J. Segura, 1992, *The mental health needs of well adolescents in families with AIDS,* New York: Human Resources Administration.

14. See C. A. Mellins and A. A. Ehrhardt, 1994, Families affected by pediatric acquired immunodeficiency syndrome: Sources of stress and coping, *Journal of Developmental and Behavioral Pediatrics* 15 (3): S54–S60 (June supplement). The authors found that although more than 50 percent of HIV-infected children included professionals in their support networks, uninfected siblings primarily relied on themselves.

15. Fanos and Wiener also document school difficulties among siblings of HIV-infected children, see note 9 above.

16. Rotheram-Borus and Draimin, see note 8 above.

17. Lamping, D. L., et al., 1991, HIV-related mental health distress in persons with HIV infection, caregivers, and family members/significant others: Results of a cross-Canada survey, *International Conference on AIDS,* 4050.

18. It may be that teens who are not ready to talk about their AIDS-related losses directly might be ready to talk about some other difficult or changing aspect of their lives that is related to the loss. It may, therefore, be preferable initially to organize generic groups that address change or difficulties in general. Youths who are ready can move on into groups that are loss-specific. A number of teen theater groups in New York have been organized specifically to give young people an opportunity to express ideas and feelings about loss creatively, and to share their experience and message with other youths.

19. The Omnibus Budget Reconciliation Act of 1993 (P.L. 103–66) permanently authorized the Independent Living Program, a part of Title IV-E of the Social Security Act. The act requires states to integrate independent living programs into their foster care systems. At state option, this program can be extended to include youths ages seventeen to twenty-one who were formerly in foster care. It also requires that case plans for foster children older than sixteen who will neither be returned to their families nor adopted include such independent living services as help completing high school or vocational programs, career planning, counseling, training in budgeting, help obtaining housing, and assistance with skills for self-sufficiency. Matching federal funds are provided to help establish and operate these programs, though no money is provided for residential or shelter services.

Chapter 6

Children and AIDS in a Multicultural Perspective

NORA ELLEN GROCE

Ethnic and minority communities are increasingly harmed by HIV disease. Poverty, isolation, and unequal access to health education and care, as well as the current epidemic of drug use in some segments of these communities, place many ethnic and minority individuals at increased risk.[1] Public health campaigns on HIV disease have been slow to reach these communities, and only recently have culturally appropriate initiatives been instituted in earnest.[2]

Too often our medical, legal, social service, and educational systems assume that all families with HIV disease need similar types of services and that all will make similar decisions regarding the care of children left orphaned. But culture plays a large part in how one views family, community, and the future. Unfortunately, our current institutional systems often lack the flexibility to permit decision making based on cultural and social values that differ from the "American norm."

There are many dimensions to these cultural differences. How do specific ethnic or minority groups differ in their definition of *family*? What role does the ethnic and minority community play in supporting families and children in times of crisis, and how can these support systems be better utilized? How do members of specific ethnic and minority groups conceptualize a child's physical and mental health needs? How does a specific ethnic or minority group explain sickness in general and AIDS in particular in the context of their broader belief systems? How does a particular cultural group conceptualize a child's understanding of death and grieving? What are the social support systems brought into play to help children through this period? Are they adequate? Where—if anywhere—do members of these communities see a role for health care professionals, mental health services, and the social work and foster care systems? How do these tie into more traditional medical and support networks? These issues are of concern because programs that are culturally sensitive will better serve families and children from communities of color and because culturally sensitive programs best ensure good compliance from these families.

HIV Disease and Family Support

Under United States law and custom, a family is assumed to be composed of a father, a mother, and a child or children—the "nuclear" family. Although other relatives such as grandparents, aunts, uncles, and cousins are considered family in the broad sense, they play no official or legal part in decision making, save in exceptional situations.

Many cultures, however, place emphasis not on the isolated nuclear family, but on the extended family. Grandparents, aunts, uncles and cousins, great-uncles and great-aunts (in some cultures even godparents and close family friends) all are considered part of an inner circle—a group of people who share the responsibility for providing legal, economic, and emotional support to children, especially when more immediate family members are unable to do so.[3] Differences between nuclear and extended family systems are illustrated by their respective resolutions of two issues of particular significance to families affected by HIV: Who in the family makes decisions for the present and future well-being of children, and who takes care of a child should parents be unable to keep the child at home?

Decision-Making Responsibility

The first issue, decision making, underscores significant cultural differences in assumptions about the individual and the family. In the United States, parents, even very young parents, are responsible for medical and custodial decisions involving their children. This exclusive locus of responsibility is far from universal. In many Asian-American and Native American households, for example, wisdom is assumed to come with age, and parents well into their twenties and thirties are considered too young to make important decisions without family discussion. Those working with such families will find it much more productive to allow parents to be joined by other family members in meetings and conferences whenever important decisions need to be made.[4]

In the Hispanic and Arabic-American communities, among others, the father (or if no father is present, the grandfather or uncle) makes major decisions on behalf of the child. Mothers may be reluctant to make decisions alone. For some women, this reluctance reflects acceptance of traditional gender roles; others fear displeasing a husband or boyfriend; still others may fear real and significant sanctions from male family members.[5]

Caring for Children

In some communities, the pattern of caring for children outside the nuclear family is already established and may represent a strength that can be built upon should a parent become incapacitated or die.[6] In the Hispanic community, for example, distant cousins and even unrelated individuals such as godparents and close family friends ("fictive kin") may be considered, and may consider themselves, active members of the family unit. These extended family members are often overlooked as resources.[7] Many urban-based African-American parents, concerned for their older children's safety and education, have traditionally sent them "back home" to the rural South for extended periods of time. The hope is that these children, raised by a grandparent or other relative, will be in a safe, supportive community with strong ties to the extended family and the church. It is not uncommon for a young teenaged boy who is beginning to get into trouble or to "run with the wrong crowd" to be sent south by anxious parents.

These long-established patterns are real strengths and are already being used when relatives become concerned about child neglect or abuse, drugs, or violence. In these situations, parents usually are not asked but rather told by their families that the children are being removed. Formal custody is not usually transferred, however, and the mechanics of providing ongoing support, financial assistance, and medical and mental health services are often complex.[8] Problems may be compounded when the relative who has taken responsibility for the child lives outside the jurisdiction of the city or state agency that has previously provided services for the family affected by HIV disease.

As the AIDS epidemic sweeps through ethnic and minority communities and the social problems of drugs, violence, and incarceration make significant destructive inroads on populations of young adults, older extended family members may be called upon to care for a number of young relatives. Grandparents, living on small pensions or a social security check, may find themselves caring for several grandchildren, some of whom may also be infected with HIV. In addition to helping with child care, these members of the extended family will often be providing care for the sick adult. The poorer the family and the more limited the community medical services, the more likely it will be that the immediate and extended family will be called upon to provide the bulk of the nursing care that the sick adult needs.[9]

Those living in ethnic and minority communities both in remote rural areas and in inner cities are more likely than many other Americans to receive health care at busy and understaffed public hospitals and clinics. Lack of health insurance contributes to this problem for many. Individuals who must use publicly funded clinics often wait until they are quite ill before seeking medical care. Furthermore, because of tight budgets and overworked staffs, many who test positive for HIV will receive less information about their diagnosis and be offered limited treatment options, social services, and mental health support programs.[10]

For many ethnic and minority families, taking care of a sick relative or that relative's child is considered to be an inescapable familial obligation, no matter how heavy the burden. As a result, children whose parents have HIV disease and limited access to health care may wind up caring for ailing parents for extended periods, and these parents may be in crisis before outside help is sought.[11] Even when these children are sent to live with relatives, much of the family's attention will still center on their seriously ill parents. Support, with special attention to the children, should be offered to these committed families.

Just as the extended family supports the individual, so the ethnic and minority community supports the extended family. Psychological, physical, and financial support are provided by many parts of the ethnic and minority community: churches, civic and fraternal organizations, societies, and social clubs.[12]

This trust and dependence on community support networks may be accompanied by an active distrust of formal medical and social services.[13] In particular, families from ethnic and minority communities often resist the intrusion of social service agencies.[14] They fear both that agencies may remove the children and place them in foster care outside the family, and that children may be placed outside the ethnic group. In all cultures, the family is seen as an ongoing link with past and future. Relatives fear that children placed in the foster care system will grow up with no knowledge of, or pride in, their family's heritage. In cultures where one's perception of the world is closely tied to one's sense of family, this is particularly alarming.

Separation of siblings in foster care is also a grave concern.[15] Among many groups, such as Asian-Americans and Hispanics, siblings have a significance beyond that understood in the Anglo-American community. It is only one's closest relatives—one's brothers or sisters—on whom one can really rely. To go out into the world without a brother or sister is to be truly alone. The idea of breaking up a family and placing children separately, perhaps permanently, in foster homes, concerns members of extended families and communities not just because these children will be separated from their current support system but also because they may grow distant from those who, according to custom, should provide their most essential support systems as adults.

Coupled with fears of placement outside the family is the fear of placement outside the ethnic group. Some communities fear that African-American, Native American/Pacific Islander, Asian-American, or Hispanic children raised in white foster care families will grow up at best distant from, and at worst without knowledge of or a sense of pride in their own heritages. As the number of children orphaned by AIDS swells and relatively few foster homes of color are available, however, this problem will not be easily rectified. Concerted efforts are necessary to recruit foster families within ethnic and minority communities.[16]

United States immigration policy, which excludes people who are infected by HIV, provides further reason to shun assistance from social service agencies. Recent immigrants may fear deportation should "the authorities" find out about their condition. Illegal aliens are at still greater risk.[17] Deportation back to a country with virtually no affordable medical care or social services for the HIV-infected immigrants or their HIV-infected child is a terrifying prospect. For such families, fear of outside authorities may far exceed fear about the declining health of a family member infected by HIV. Children in such families live not only with the burden of their parent's illness but with the fear that assistance and support may bring with it deportation and separation from their current family, friends, homes, and schools.

Acculturation and the Community

Maintaining an ethnic identity in the face of dominant and often dominating American society is a challenge, and not all members of any community agree on what aspects of American culture to adopt and what to leave alone. Older members of most ethnic and minority communities tend to adhere to more traditional concepts. Young adults, particularly those who have grown up in the United States, may rely little on traditional values. Acculturated to modern American life, these young adults may be far more influenced by the popular media than by traditional community beliefs. Their views on heritage, religion, education, and the obligations to distant family members may be significantly different from those of their parents and grandparents. Indeed, many young adults may reject traditional beliefs and values outright and may raise their children in a way pointedly similar to that of the American mainstream.

When an acculturated young adult becomes infected with HIV disease, more traditional family members may believe (whether true or not) that the infected relative placed himself or herself at risk for disease by straying from the old ways—using drugs, having sex outside (or instead of) marriage, or socializing with others outside the traditional culture. Acculturated parents with HIV disease may be more willing than are their extended families to rely on outside support services.[18] Public health nurses, home health aides, and social workers may provide welcome support for the ailing parent, though the extended family views them as unwelcome visitors interfering with private family politics. Older family members, in particular, may see such outside support services as yet another affront to their traditional values perpetuated by a child who has already strayed too far into mainstream American culture. Older, more traditional relatives may oppose mental health and counseling services in particular, though they may be sorely needed and desired by more acculturated dying parents and affected children.

Cultural Perceptions of Life, Death, and AIDS

All groups have ideas about the meaning of disease, life, and death. Indeed, these shared sets of beliefs, including beliefs about illness, help to define specific distinct sociocultural groups. Although most Americans have heard that AIDS is caused by a virus, the infection of a specific individual is often cause for cultural interpretation.[19] Members of a culture may believe that AIDS represents a punishment for sin, a curse, or a test from God or the gods of one's faith or the faith of one's family. When the illness is believed to have been acquired by a serious breach of widely held community values, the sympathy and support given to an infected individual may be diminished, or may be offered with a judgmental tone.

Cultural differences exist not only in theories of disease causation, but also in the response to disease. Although younger and more acculturated members of a family may turn to physicians and hospitals to maintain health for as long as possible, older and less acculturated members of many communities may also attempt to involve traditional healers and spiritualists.[20] These different approaches may cause friction within the family, but in some cases traditional healers may provide psychological and/or physical treatments that may make patients (or their families) more comfortable.[21] Medical personnel should encourage families to use traditional medical systems when some benefit seems to be derived (or at least no harm done).

Sickness and the "Sick Role"

All cultures have "appropriate" ways of being sick and appropriate ways for families to care for someone who is sick. Anglo-American culture stresses independence and assumes that individuals who are sick, particularly those who are seriously ill, will want to maintain their independence for as long as possible. But cultures that stress family interdependence, such as Hispanic or African-American families, view sickness as a time for the family to draw closer.[22] The sick are not to be left alone; relatives may mount efforts to provide around-the-clock care. Indeed, many members of ethnic and minority groups interpret the American insistence on independence when one is seriously ill as showing a lack of concern and a cold indifference to family responsibilities.[23]

Health care and social service professionals who encourage adults with HIV disease to maintain their independence may be perceived as a threat, attempting to drive a wedge between the older generation and their more acculturated sick offspring just when these young people are believed to be in greatest need of family support and encouragement. In addition, because many ethnic and minority communities closely monitor the care given to the sick and elderly, a family may be particularly concerned about being disgraced or dishonored in the eyes of the community by "abandoning" a sick relative.

The culturally defined "sick role" is often gender specific, with males, especially male heads of household and oldest sons, the recipients of a disproportionate amount of nursing care. Women, especially younger women, are less likely to be granted the same amount of support. This is particularly true for young adult women, who are expected to care for husbands or boyfriends, aging parents, and children as well as run a household and often maintain a job to add to the family income. When family members are infected with HIV, these women are also expected to take on the role of nursing husband or boyfriend and sick children, even while the women may themselves be beginning to show the ravages of the disease. In these instances, women may neglect or significantly delay their own care, much to their own detriment.[24]

HIV disease places immense and unique burdens on the traditional practice whereby family members provide around-the-clock care for the sick. Intensive nursing care and support for a sick family member works well for short-term illnesses. But patients with HIV disease can live for months or years while families scramble to provide assistance and still carry on with the rest of their lives.

The role that children, particularly older children, are expected to assume in caring for increasingly ill parents and surviving siblings is of particular concern. Children, even young children, may be expected to function as primary caregivers for ailing parents, especially if other relatives live far away.[25] This burden may be great, particularly on older children and teenagers. Traditional families may press far more acculturated teenagers and young adults to take over responsibilities for younger siblings. A daughter, in particular, may be kept home from school to be a nurse, a housekeeper, and a caretaker for younger siblings. A young man may be expected to drop out of high school or come home from college to become the breadwinner so the family can afford to stay together. Professionals working with these families need to provide support for these older teenagers and young adults so they can balance their own aspirations with their sense of responsibility for younger siblings.

Cultural Interpretations of Death and Childhood Grieving

Cultures provide members with shared beliefs not only about the cause and consequences of illness, but also about the meaning of death and the appropriate way to express grief and loss. The manner in which children can express sadness over the declining health or death of parents or siblings will, in part, be culturally determined.[26]

Not all cultures envision the needs of individuals, particularly the mental health needs of children, in the same way as middle-class Anglo-Americans might. In some cultures, children, even older children, are not considered mature enough to understand issues of life and death. Consequently, a child will receive no explanation if a parent or sibling becomes sick with AIDS. The child may not be told what to expect even if he or she carries the virus. When children are supposed to "be seen and not heard," there is often little forum for them to express fear, anger, sadness, or despair. Counseling in many ethnic/minority communities is scorned, particularly for children, and seen as an admission that someone is "crazy"—a major impediment to service for many children who desperately need help.[27]

Long-term mourning and continuing adjustments—as conceptualized by child psychologists—are not, in some cultures, considered normal parts of childhood. Children who fail to adjust quickly to the death of a parent or sibling are thought to be overly sensitive. The surviving parent or the grandparent caring for such a child may be criticized by other members of the community for "coddling" or "spoiling" the child. At the same time, many communities have strong traditional support systems that may be enlisted by formal service systems far more frequently to assist children and their families touched by HIV disease. Community and religious leaders, respected teachers and elders, and community and church groups that already function as support networks can be utilized far more regularly and far more effectively.[28]

Recommendations for Culturally Sensitive Approaches for Children and Families Coping with HIV Disease

Simply labeling a policy or program "culturally sensitive" or "culturally competent" does not necessarily make it so. To be successful, programs, policies, and outreach efforts must make a real difference to the health, well-being, and peace of mind of children and families in these communities. To that end, the following recommendations are offered to assist in developing HIV-related programs in our ethnically diverse communities:

• When parents and/or children who have the HIV virus are members of an extended family network, this extended family should be included in the care and decision-making process. The individual with HIV disease is the best judge of who is and who is not important in the decision-making process. When such individuals request that extended family be included in discussions or plans, their wishes should, to the fullest extent possible, be honored.

• A number of traditional support networks already exist in ethnic and minority communities, including churches, synagogues, and mosques, as well as fraternal organizations, clubs, and societies. They represent a resource that might be used more effectively both in AIDS prevention campaigns and in caring for adults and children affected by the disease. The agencies serving HIV-infected individuals and families need to increase their efforts to target these support networks and establish cooperative working relationships with them.

• Children need forums in which to express their fears and concerns, as well as their hopes and dreams. There are some culturally accepted forums—Sunday school, community groups, and ethnic clubs, for example—where children regularly speak about important issues in their lives. Adults who direct and work in these organizations should be provided with better information about how best to help and work with children affected by HIV disease.

• Culturally appropriate community outreach efforts should be encouraged, and community-based sources of information, including ethnic and foreign-language newspapers, radio, and television, should be more effectively used in both AIDS education and HIV support efforts.

• Ethnic and minority groups, like other communities, often maintain a number of negative stereotypes about HIV disease. Confronting negative stereotypes about AIDS in these communities is essential, and the leadership of these communities must be enlisted in this endeavor.[29]

• Communities of color must be included in the development of HIV-related policy and programs from the outset, not simply asked to evaluate programs and policies developed by others. Otherwise, well-intentioned programs will be met with caution. Caution and distrust of program and policy planning are substantial barriers to serving communities of color.[30] This distrust has firm roots in histories of discrimination, insufficient regard for the health of people of color, and inappropriate scientific experimentation on these populations. Caution also reflects concern within these communities about the loss of tradition—tradition that represents an important source of strength for many individuals, families, and communities as they confront the AIDS epidemic.

Notes

1. *Ethnicity* and *minority* are very general terms that must be used with some caution. Ethnicity generally applies to groups with a shared cultural heritage, such as Latin Americans or Southeast Asians. Minority refers to a group distinguished on the basis of race, such as African-Americans. Both terms are imprecise and present problems. African-Americans, for example, are distinguished not only by race but also by a shared heritage and a distinct culture. West Indians, although they also trace their heritage to Africa, do not generally consider themselves part of the African-American community.

Moreover, within each of these categories are many distinct subgroups based on regional, socioeconomic, educational, and social affiliations. For example, a Hispanic individual can come from one of more than twenty national cultures. The family of an African-American college professor with HIV disease will most likely have different social, educational, and economic concerns than the family of a young mother in an inner-city housing project. Because national statistics use only the broadest of categories, they mask the fact that infection rates are strikingly different among subgroups. (Morales, J., and M. Bok, 1992, *Multicultural human services for AIDS treatment and prevention*, Binghamton, N.Y.: Haworth Press; Peruga, A., and M. Rivo, 1992, Racial differences in AIDS knowledge among adults, *AIDS Education and Prevention* 4 (1): 52–60.) For example, AIDS prevalence is markedly different between Koreans and Filipinos, even though both are grouped together under the single category Asian-American/Pacific Islanders. (National Minority AIDS Council, 1992, *The impact on communities of color: A blueprint for the nineties*, Washington, D.C.: National Minority AIDS Council.) Finally, while ethnic or minority affiliation may help in understanding how best to support families and children in crisis, no two individuals or two families are alike. Ethnic or minority status is not, in itself, a diagnostic category.

2. National Commission on AIDS, 1992, *The challenge of HIV/AIDS in communities of color*, Maryland: National Commission on AIDS; Diaz, T., et al., 1993, AIDS trends among Hispanics in the United States, *American Journal of Public Health* 83 (4): 504–509; National Center for Health Statistics, 1991, *AIDS knowledge and attitudes of black Americans: United States, 1990*, Hyattsville, Md.: U.S. Dept. of Health and Human Services, Public Health Service, CDC; National Center for Health Statistics, 1991, *AIDS knowledge and attitudes of Hispanic Americans: United States, 1990*, Hyattsville, Md.: U.S. Dept. of Health and Human Services, Public Health Service, CDC; National Minority AIDS Council, see note 1 above.

3. Richardson, L., 1993, Adoptions that lack papers, not purpose, *New York Times*, November 23, 1993; Vidal, C., 1988, Godparenting among Hispanic Americans, *Child Welfare* 67 (5): 453–459.

4. Galanti, G., 1991, *Caring for patients from different cultures: Case studies from American hospitals*, Philadelphia: University of Pennsylvania Press; Gross, N., and K. Zola, 1993, Multiculturalism, chronic illness, and disability, *Pediatrics* 91 (5): 1048–1055; Lynch, E., and M. Hanson, 1992, *Developing cross-cultural competence: A guide for working with young children and their families*, Baltimore: Paul Brooks.

5. Foster, P., et al., 1993, An Africentric model for AIDS education, prevention, and psychological services within the African-American community, *Journal of Black Psychology* 19 (2): 123–141; Kalichman, S., et al., 1993, Culturally tailored HIV-AIDS risk-reduction messages targeted to African-American urban women: Impact of risk sensitization and risk reduction, *Journal of Consulting and Clinical Psychology* 61 (2): 291–295.

6. Gray, S., and L. Nybell, 1990, Issues in African-American family preservation, *Child Welfare* 69 (6): 513–523; Scott, J., and A. Black, 1989, Deep structures of African-American family life: Female and male kin networks, *Western Journal of Black Studies* 13 (1): 17–24; Lynch and Hanson, see note 4 above.

7. Vidal, see note 3 above.

8. Hill, R., 1977, *Informal adoption among black families*, Washington, D.C.: National Urban League; Richardson, see note 3 above.

9. Lester, C., and L. Saxxon, 1988, AIDS in the black community: The plague, the politics, the people, *Death Studies* 12 (5–6): 563–571; Morales and Bok, see note 1 above; National Minority AIDS Council, see note 1 above.

10. National Commission on AIDS, see note 2 above; Lester and Saxxon, see note 9 above; Morales and Bok, see note 1 above; National Minority AIDS Council, see note 1 above.

11. National Center for Health Statistics, report on Hispanic Americans, see note 2 above.

12. Cancela, V., and A. McDowell, 1992, AIDS: Health care intervention models for communities of color, in Morales and Bok, see note 1 above, 107–119; Galanti, see note 4 above; Lester and Saxxon, see note 9 above.

13. Dalton, H., 1989, AIDS in blackface, *Daedalus* 118 (3): 205–227; Quimby, E., 1993, Obstacles to reducing AIDS among African-Americans, *Journal of Black Psychology* 19 (2): 215–222; Thomas, S., and S. Quinn, 1991, The Tuskegee syphilis study, 1932 to 1972: Implications for HIV education and AIDS risk reduction programs in the black community, *American Journal of Public Health* 81 (11): 1298–1305; Lester and Saxxon, see note 9 above.

14. Cancela and McDowell, see note 12 above; Gross and Zola, see note 4 above; Horsjsi, C., B. Craig, and J. Pablo, 1992, Reactions by Native American parents to child protection agencies: Culture and community factors, *Child Welfare* 71 (4): 329–342; National Minority AIDS Council, see note 1 above; Mellins, C. A., and A. A. Ehrhardt, 1994, Families affected by pediatric acquired immunodeficiency syndrome: Sources of stress and coping, *Journal of Developmental and Behavioral Pediatrics* 15 (3): S54–S60 (June supplement).

15. For a discussion of the importance of sibling bonds see J. Fanos and L. Wiener, 1994, Tomorrow's survivors: Siblings of human immunodeficiency virus-infected children, *Journal of Developmental and Behavioral Pediatrics* 15 (3): S43–S48 (June supplement); K. Siegel and E. Gorey, 1994, Childhood bereavement due to parental death from acquired immunodeficiency syndrome, *Journal of Developmental and Behavioral Pediatrics* 15 (3): S66–S70 (June supplement).

16. Gray and Nybell, see note 6 above; Horsjsi, Craig, and Pablo, see note 14 above; Scott and Black, see note 6 above.

17. Gross and Zola, see note 4 above; National Center for Health Statistics, see note 2 above (both studies).

18. Brancho de Carpio, A., F. Carpio-Cedrano, and L. Anderson, 1990, Hispanic families learning and teaching about AIDS, *Journal of Behavioral Sciences* 12 (2): 165–176; Campos, A., 1988, A Puerto Rican perspective on counselling, *Counselling and Treating People of Color* 1 (1): 2; Peruga and Rivo, see note 1 above.

19. Galanti, see note 4 above; Lynch and Hanson, see note 4 above; National Center for Health Statistics, see note 2 above (both studies).

20. Flaskerud, J., and C. Rush, 1989, AIDS and traditional health beliefs and practices of black women, *Nursing Research* 38 (4): 210–215; McCallum, D., J. Esser-Stuart, J. Howell, and D. Klemmach, 1992, AIDS: Assessing African-American knowledge and attitudes for community education programs, in Morales and Bok, see note 1 above.

21. Gross and Zola, see note 4 above.

22. Brancho de Carpio, Carpio-Cedrano, and Anderson, see note 18 above; Gross and Zola, see note 4 above; Morales and Bok, see note 1 above.

23. McDonell, J., N. Abell, and J. Miller, 1991, Family members' willingness to care for people with AIDS: A psychosocial assessment model, *Social Work* 36 (1): 43–53; Cancela and McDowell, see note 12 above.

24. Foster et al., see note 5 above; Morales and Bok, see note 1 above; National Minority AIDS Council, see note 1 above.

25. Galanti, see note 4 above; Lynch and Hanson, see note 4 above; National Minority AIDS Council, see note 1 above.

26. Lynch and Hanson, see note 4 above.

27. Campos, see note 18 above; Cancela and McDowell, see note 12 above; Foster et al., see note 5 above.

28. McCallum et al., see note 20 above; National Minority AIDS Council, see note 1 above; Quimby, E., see note 13 above.

29. Kalichman et al., see note 5 above; National Minority AIDS Council, see note 1 above.

30. Dalton, see note 13 above; Horsjsi, Craig, and Pablo, see note 14 above; Lester and Saxxon, see note 9 above; Thomas and Quinn, see note 13 above.

Chapter 7

What Can We Learn from Children of War?

ROBERTA J. APFEL AND CYNTHIA J. TELINGATOR

The twentieth century has been a time of great paradox for children. More than ever, we have become aware of their special emotional, physical, and developmental needs, their vulnerabilities, and the need to protect them from exploitation in the labor force. We assert their rights to education, nutrition, and loving parental adults. On the other hand, children have been exposed to unprecedented warfare and violence that has profoundly and negatively affected them. At the close of this century, though we profess concern for children, we still debate whether the United States will ratify the United Nations Declaration on the Rights of Children, at what age—twelve years, fifteen, eighteen?—it is all right for children to become soldiers, and how to help the millions of children who are orphans, refugees, or otherwise unaccompanied minors.

Some children in the United States suffer losses and an early exposure to violence that parallel the experience of children and adolescents from war zones in other countries. Two areas of childhood experience in which there are some specific and powerful parallels are war and AIDS. Because children in war have been studied for over fifty years—some now followed to adulthood—much has been learned about the impact of the war experience on their development. This chapter explores what we have learned from these survivors and applies these findings to the particular experience of children who are living with the impact of the AIDS epidemic. Children who are survivors of the AIDS epidemic experience an economic and cultural devastation that can be similar to that of children who witness their world systematically eradicated by war. In many families the virus has infected multiple family members and will devastate the family, much as war can decimate families. But regardless of what these groups of children share, each child is alone— each has an individual story and tragedy.

Other chapters have addressed the complicated task faced by children and teenagers living in families with HIV disease. These children face an enemy that resides within and has no face, nor foreign ethnicity or culture. The enemy is a virus that has invaded the body of people they love. By discussing the experience of children in war in counterpoint with presentations about children affected by AIDS, we hope to elucidate issues that are important to all caregivers working with these children. Our vantage point as psychiatrist clinicians enables us to see the inner pain of one child and family at a time, a microcosm of the larger problem faced by so many children.

Common Themes

Certain themes are repeatedly heard from children who are or have been in conditions of great hardship. These themes cross cultures and locations, specific experiences, and even the age and the developmental level of the child.

Shame and Responsibility

Before the age of puberty (consonant with their neurophysiological and cognitive development), children tend to see themselves as responsible for events around them.[1] When a young child wishes that something bad would happen to another and then learns that the person has had an accident, the child feels magically responsible, as if the wish itself was powerful enough to cause the harm. This is especially true for children living with illness or violence; they become frightened of their own imagined power and feel that the plight of others is their fault. They sense that they are different from their peers whom they would like to resemble, and they feel alone and ashamed. Children believe that they should have the ability to change situations. When they cannot effect a desired change, they often feel guilty and depressed. Their feelings are expressed in ways that are consistent with gender, developmental age, culture, and social constraints. Some child survivors of the Holocaust, interviewed fifty years later, report that they felt they were perhaps responsible for the tension within the family and for what happened to them and their families.[2] Though adults now, they have never fully dismissed their guilty belief. So, too, do children with parents infected by HIV express feelings of personal responsibility for their parents' plight (see, for example, the March 30 entry of Onivea's journal, reprinted in this volume).

Keeping Secrets and Feeling Isolated

Children living under great hardship are often not told the nature of the problems in a way appropriate to their age and developmental stage. Or they may elect to be silent because of their shame and fear of being stigmatized. In some families, a parent will make a disclosure but then request that the child maintain the secret to protect the child and family from further ostracism. The shroud of secrecy serves to further separate the growing child from his or her own perceptions and feelings and from others, including those who might be able to provide help. The theme of silence predominates in Holocaust literature. Dan Bar-On has shown the common burden of silence for the children whose parents were Nazis during World War II and for the children whose parents were victims of that war.[3] Fifty years after the war, the experience of living with silence has been a source of bonding for these two once-antagonistic groups. One of the darkest secrets children in such situations share is the continuing pain of the traumatic experience decades after the event, even for those whose lives appear to be successful and intact. We have learned that breaking the silence, finding others who know the same hidden anguish, can be healing. This general insight needs to be applied individually for each child in each family affected by AIDS.

Isolation, both emotional and social, can result from any significant disruption in life. Whether war occurs once within a short span of time or chronically over one's whole childhood, there are inevitable upheavals, with multiple losses of loved ones, homes, neighborhoods, schools, familiar flora and fauna, and language. Even for children who appear to make an excellent adjustment to disruptions in their family, there is a sense of isolation from the mainstream in their society. They may not ever feel that they fully belong. This isolation exists even for children who have come as refugees in the best of circumstances—with intact family and some financial security. A child may begin to feel less marginal in one situation and then, when experiencing another loss or even a developmental milestone, may feel quite isolated again. This pattern is equally true for children coping with HIV in their families. Each deterioration in the condition of an infected parent makes the child feel more isolated, because each such change is experienced as a loss.

Multiple Losses

Children of war and children of AIDS typically experience multiple losses. Rarely is there only a transient exposure to a single wartime experience, but even children so affected are influenced by the events and haunted for a lifetime. More commonly children of war suffer losses of family, pets, and home, as well as the experience of poverty, dislocation, starvation, loss of identity, loss of childhood, and a loss of a trusted network of care providers. Abandonment by a parent is the loss children fear the most. Even temporary separations can be frightening for young children, who may fear that the loss will be total and permanent. Fantasies of desertion are especially prevalent in very young children who are totally dependent on parents, and even these fantasies can be terrifying. When reality conforms to the child's worst fear—when a parent *does* disappear forever, either in war or because of AIDS—the emotional consequences are disastrous.

We have learned that children who do best in wartime situations are those whose mothers organize themselves to protect them. Children who stayed with their mothers during the London blitz did better than those sent to safety in the country.[4] More recently in strife-torn Lebanon, the mother's behavior was the main predictor of a child's mental health.[5] When there are no mothers or mother figures to buffer the child from the threatening situation, however—for example, when a child's mother is the one infected by HIV—the child will suffer the most.

Some children may sustain many losses but still manage to remain connected to a parent in fantasy or through linking objects that remind the child of the parent in a concrete way. Note, for example, how Onivea keeps a relationship alive with her departed mother by writing letters to her. A boy in a Tunis orphanage provided another example. He had a scar on his foot from a burn suffered in his grandmother's house. He used the scar as a link to a lost home and parent and used the foot to kick and become a star soccer player.[6]

We know from studying children in war that the experience of multiple losses may leave one vulnerable to loss and disruption later in life.[7] Such children may become so cynical and numb that they fail to connect with or trust any person in their later lives. Even those who have acknowledged their losses may not be able to fully grieve for many years, if ever, and may have symptoms in body and/or behavior of frozen grief. Such frozen or pathological grief is expressed in fatigue (it takes a lot of energy to defend against grief), somatic symptoms, inner deadness, and a loss of interest in people and things.[8] The child—or the adult who suffered the losses as a child—may not show the expected sadness, dejection, or unhappiness usually associated with the loss of loved ones. He or she may express a lifelong dissatisfaction, emptiness, and yearning that can never be filled by anyone. We can anticipate that children who suffer multiple AIDS-related losses will be at least equally vulnerable.

Moral Compromise

Moral compromise is reported by child survivors of war and is also seen among children in AIDS families. The shame associated with what they have seen, and with what they may have had to do to survive, is carried as a further scar, as something that may further isolate them from others. Survivors of the Holocaust were especially eager, upon their release from concentration camps, to reestablish a moral order, something they had lived without for years. Some report that they insisted on working and paying for food and haircuts even when those things were provided free. Similarly, a child whose mother has AIDS may have seen the mother behave in ways that are not legal or ethical by society's standards, as in the following case. The surviving child may feel compelled to right the order later in life.

> Charlene was discovered by staff members to be selling her pain medication. Although she had said she was not a drug user and not "seeing" her ex-boyfriend, a drug dealer, and although she needed the Percodan for her pain, she sold the pills for money. This set a terrible example, she realized, for her eight-year-old daughter, for whom she wanted a better, more honest life than she herself had led. When we discovered that her reason for selling the medication was to pay for manicures for herself and her daughter, it seemed that Charlene had made a choice with its own morality. Perhaps the daughter in future years could use her fingernails as a linking object to her lost mother. She might remember her mother's choice for life and beauty, and her willingness to forgo pain medication to share such an experience with her daughter before she died.

Providing Settings That Maximize a Child's Resilience

Children who have the luck to survive war usually share certain characteristics of general intellectual and affective competence, particularly the ability to engage the adults around them and thus obtain nurture; the ability to nurture others (caring for younger children, for example); and a rich fantasy life that gives some sustaining purpose, image, or goal to keep them going. Our work with children of war has also shown that connections with peers who have sustained similar losses seem crucial to survival.[9] Indeed, we have learned that some children do better in group homes than in foster care after losing parents in a disaster. Vamik Volkan found that orphans from Sabra and Shattila functioned well in the Tunis orphanage until he tried to interview them one on one. When the peer group was separated, several children rapidly decompensated in a terrified, psychotic regression. For these children, an attachment to an individual was too threatening, the potential for loss too great. While in a group, the children felt supported and attached to many people rather than vulnerable to the loss of another significant person. Schools can be ideal places for focused healing because they are normative environments for peers. Manuals for teachers working with children in war zones explain how to identify problems and how the school curriculum can be used for helping the child.[10]

These lessons drawn from children in situations of war have major implications for children affected by AIDS. The child welfare system has been eager to replicate for most children the ideal of a family home, with parents and a few other children. But a new home can rarely compare favorably to the home that the child lost, or to the one that the child fantasizes. We should not assume that group homes are inappropriate for all children. For older children they may provide a more therapeutic environment than foster homes. We should also be developing school curricula that acknowledge the impact of this epidemic on the lives of so many children and that provide the affected children with settings in which they can maximize their own individual resilient capacities. We can help families by attempting to make optimal arrangements for each child, with an emphasis on early interventions based on the child's individual needs.

Giving Voice to Trauma

The trauma of war can be ameliorated for children. We have learned that children can be helped to cope by getting them together in groups; by encouraging creative and nonverbal expressions such as art, dance, and theater (both because some of the trauma has been unspeakable and because some of the children are too young to verbalize); and by getting the children to talk with a reliable, trusted adult. The use of culturally sensitive material, including crafts, music, and language, has the added benefit of reconnecting the child to a culture that seems to have been lost to him or her. Schools and community organizations play crucial roles, as do elders from the same culture. Such elders—either actual or surrogate grandparents—can be links to the past and provide a sense of continuity and longevity. In interviewing Palestinian children we learned how grandmothers' stories of the past have helped sustain children during war:

> With his father imprisoned, Ahmed, by age twelve, was already frustrated with curfews, the presence of soldiers, and school closings. His paternal grandmother shared his loss and concern for his father and the daily turmoil. She told him stories about when she was his age, and about how things got better and worse over many years. She sang him traditional Palestinian songs and cooked his father's favorite food. She also showed him a house key she kept from when she was twelve, a time when her family had to move during a war. The key was her symbol of hope and link to her past. Ahmed's time with his grandmother gave him knowledge of someone else's childhood hardship and helped him to learn that one could still live a long, hopeful, and fulfilling life.

Gilbert Kliman, who has studied bereavement among children in foster care, developed a workbook that younger children (ages three to eleven) can complete with a foster parent, teacher, or therapist, and that older children can work on independently. This book documents a past for the child—including birth parents and previous home and life—and thereby gives the child a book in which he or she is the hero of a life story. Kliman has found that foster children who do this workbook and bond with their foster parents in the process of completing it are unlikely to require further foster home placements.[11]

These lessons suggest that in working with children from AIDS-affected families, we must maintain and build connections to their cultural roots and supports, to church, neighborhood, homeland, and family. We must not compound their losses unnecessarily by separating them from these sources of strength.

Caretakers' Challenges

Childhood survivors of the Holocaust rarely seek psychiatric treatment, and those who do usually come for help late in life or, inadvertently, for something else. They do not seek care because they expressly wish not to be stigmatized further as psychiatric patients, to be diagnosed and categorized as they were during the war. Professionals to whom these survivors come for help are not usually people who have shared the experience. The surviving child of war may feel that the caretaker cannot really "get it." When provided with a safe environment to tell his or her story, the child often reveals only portions at a time. The story is retold, reedited, and rewritten—consciously and unconsciously—to protect himself or herself and the caregiver as well from the overwhelming trauma of reexperiencing the story in its entirety. So, too, children in families with AIDS may assume responsibility to protect the infected parent and may decide, when in therapy, to protect the therapist. Indeed, caretakers who listen to these stories can be overwhelmed. They need support and supervision to cope with the shared sadness, pain, and feelings of helplessness.

"Burnout" among caretakers of children of war is managed through group support, through affirmation of life (dancing, singing, joking, laughing), and through diversification of work. Diversion from work is also important; it is therapeutic to take time to write and to get away, to remind oneself that the burdens can be borne, and to remember that "going under" does no one any good.[12]

These lessons about caring for the caretakers have direct implications for those who work in the AIDS war. They, too, not only hear the stories, but experience their unfolding. They get to know and to feel attached to people who will die prematurely. They find themselves mourning repeated losses and dealing both with their personal helplessness and with their general hopelessness in the face of the devastation this virus causes to individuals, families, and society. They, too, need to be supported, in all of the same ways now used to reduce burnout among caretakers of children of war.

Differences Between Children of War and Children of AIDS

The Process of Healing

Over the years, we have learned that a major way the child of war heals is by creating a new family in adult life.[13] For a child suffering family losses from AIDS, however, this way of healing is complicated by the manner in which HIV is transmitted, the very reason for the child's losses.

In HIV disease, love, sex, and intimacy are transformed to death. Parents can expose one another to HIV, and the infection can be transmitted to their children. This creates turmoil for children reaching adolescence, for AIDS has been linked with sexuality in a confusing way. Many people initially attempted to dismiss the dangers associated with this faceless enemy by naming it the "gay disease," stigmatizing and isolating it through association with a group that was already socially marginalized. Homosexual men were labeled as the enemy, with the implication that the infection was a justified retribution for "deviant" sexual behavior.

Some children, having been exposed to this attitude, may maintain the belief that anyone who contracts AIDS must have been sexually deviant, promiscuous, or otherwise deserving of the plight. Young survivors of this epidemic may perceive intimacy as potentially deadly and may either repeat the destruction by rushing into sexuality prematurely or fearfully avoid the potential healing that enduring intimate relationships might provide.

> Christine, a fifteen-year-old girl, was in repeated conflict with her mother, who is HIV infected. A family member disclosed the news of her mother's infection to others in the neighborhood, causing Christine to learn about it before her mother was ready to tell her and before she was symptomatic. Christine has been terrified, angry, and despondent since learning of her mother's diagnosis. At times she wishes she herself could be infected and stay with her mother always. She impulsively abandons friends and school to be with her mother. She repeatedly runs away and exposes herself to HIV by engaging in unprotected sex and taking drugs. She believes (as a much younger child might) that if she is infected, it will magically spare her mother; even if that sacrifice fails, Christine's death will spare her the pain of abandonment. She tries many routes to rescue her mother, promising to fulfill her mother's dream of having a house where Christine will take care of her younger siblings. If she goes to college—another fantasy of her mother's—she wonders if she

will save her mother or rather surpass her and hasten her demise.

Christine got a job to support the family, hoping that her mother's boyfriend would leave and that Christine would again be the focus of her mother's attention. Her mother countenances Christine's truancy and academic failure because her presence at home means that neither will have to bear the terror alone. Christine tries to affirm life; she fantasizes that she will get pregnant and that the baby will give its grandmother the will to live, saving her from AIDS. The mutual ambivalence about having one survive without the other was exemplified on one occasion when Christine and her mother fought viciously. Scratched by Christine, her mother displayed her bloodied arm and said, "You better wash up, because I can give you this [invisible] disease!" The intimacy and rage of this moment had the potential to take another life.

The Sense of Community

For children who lose their parents in ethnic and religious wars, the community reinforces the notion that the loss, however tragic, was for a greater cause. The community's reverence allows the child to maintain a fantasized relationship with the lost parent, so important for the survival of many children of war. Society may even take up the role of parent for these child survivors. When an Israeli soldier dies, for example, the Army takes on a parental role in both symbolic and practical ways, such as by taking the soldier's children to summer camp.[14]

In contrast, with HIV disease, there is no sense of an all-inclusive community and no ideology or purpose to which the deaths can be attributed. People with HIV disease, who come from diverse groups, many of which are already marginalized in our society (such as drug users and prostitutes), are further ostracized once infected. The response to AIDS can be different within each group, and affected groups may not even demonstrate sympathy for each other. For example, AIDS is a different disease for gay men than it is for women. Gay men mobilized and consolidated around the common enemy, AIDS. In contrast, women with AIDS are still disenfranchised, disorganized, silent, and less economically empowered.

Families living with HIV disease may feel estranged from their own religious and ethnic communities; they often hide their illness from these communities for fear of ostracism, or they may lie about the true cause of death, attributing it to cancer, for example. When a death occurs, the extended family may turn to its community for support but may still maintain a conspiracy of silence about the individual who has died for fear of further stigmatization and isolation.

To the child living in these families, this silence may come to represent something shameful associated with the loss, and the child may internalize a sense of being different and bad. Maintaining a fantasized relationship with the lost parent, so important for survival of many children of war, is complicated by the community's lack of reverence. The child, yearning for a connection with the parent may repeat the parent's own behaviors (such as drug use) and thus be exposed to a risk of contracting HIV.

Sometimes the therapist becomes the child's "community." While the child continues to mourn the lost parent, the therapist may have to bear his or her negative emotions, such as rage at abandonment, and may have to work over a long period to help the child learn that his or her anger is not powerful enough to make helping adults disappear.

> Anthony was barely six years old when his mother, sick with AIDS, arranged for him to see a therapist. She was concerned about his inability to leave her and about his habit of curling up in bed in a fetal position and sucking his thumb. We realize in retrospect that she also wanted to build a network of caretakers who could become a community for her son after her death. Many members of the extended family had already died and others were infected with HIV. Eventually, both of his parents died and the family became estranged. A family member who was to be a guardian moved out of state and never returned. Anthony could not trust that anyone would "be there" for him.
>
> His mother tried to keep her four children together in subsidized housing, which was a familiar home, but, sick and alone, it was difficult for her to maintain a household. Extended family members alternated in caring for the children, but in an inconsistent way. The association with the therapist has been Anthony's most steady and predictable relationship. Anthony knows that the therapist knew and respected his mother. He can acknowledge his deepest yearnings to the therapist and return emotionally to places that have been fraught with pain and ambivalence. He can ameliorate the losses of his parents by expressing his anger at the therapist when she is not present for a weekly session, his terror that the therapist will not return from vacation, and his relief when she returns.

Maintaining a Vision of an Idealized Parent

For many children of war, maintaining a vision of an idealized parent is not difficult; their communities revere their parents, who championed the community's cause. However, with HIV disease, the child faces two challenges in maintaining an idealized vision of a parent. First, the child watches as the parent wastes away, becomes helpless, cachectic, and even demented. Death is not sudden. It is long anticipated and can be greeted with relief—and guilt.

Second, the child cannot rely on the community to sustain the vision of the idealized dead parent because the community itself has devalued that parent. The child must then live with shame.

Some parents who are diagnosed with HIV disease may struggle, sometimes for the first time ever, to be ideal parents. Some are mobilized to the full task of parenting after the diagnosis, becoming, for an all too brief time between diagnosis and terminal illness, the kind of parents they had wished to be. Until symptoms of the illness intrude, children receive a hint of the good parents they might have had, causing further anger when the suddenly good parents can no longer fulfill that role.

> When Sandra learned of her HIV infection, she stopped using drugs and devoted herself to her eleven-year-old daughter, Sophie, and her eight-year-son, Tom, who had previously lived intermittently in foster care and with their respective fathers and grandmothers. Sandra started to attend her mother's church and reconciled her relationship with her own God-fearing mother, who agreed to take care of both children after Sandra's death. Meanwhile, Sandra told the children nothing of her illness.
>
> For about a year, the children enjoyed their mother's presence, though they resented her new boyfriend, Dan. As Sandra became sicker, she had to struggle to maintain her appearance and to continue to participate in bingo games at church. She demanded that the visiting nurses come to the house only as friends and that they never carry their medical bags, which would identify the purpose of the house call. She still did not tell Sophie about the diagnosis.
>
> Sophie devoted herself to school and found refuge away from home, getting especially attached to a teacher. Finally, one day, when Sandra felt ill and fearful of her impending death, she told Sophie to stay home from school. She instructed her daughter how to give medications and told her that she should keep silent when neighbors asked questions about whatever was happening in the home. Sophie suddenly lost her teacher and classmates, who had become her support network, but she felt she could not get angry at her mother, who was so obviously sick and weak.
>
> Tom stayed away from home and school increasingly. He grew angry at having no role to play and no attention given to him. The children were overstimulated by their mother's weakness, difficulty eating, and pain; they were given no information or steady parenting after that first year. Because of the progression of her illness Sandra could neither tend to her children nor continue to build the connection to their grandmother that she had arranged for their future. By the time Sandra died, everyone was resentful of her and angry at one another. The grandmother inherited a situation so chaotic that its repair seemed impossible.

The Sense of Time

A sense of the future and of time is very important to all children—"When I grow up . . ." and "Once upon a time, when . . ." are archetypal expressions of that fundamental concern. Losing a sense of the continuity of time is common for children of war. These children may be unable to account for whole years of life and school lost; refugee children sometimes forget their birthdays or even lose track of their birth years with no one to help mark and order the time. Once peace is reestablished, however, these children can begin new counts—the number of years since arriving in the new country or since the release from the "DP" (displaced person) camp, or even the years since the "bad old days."

Children of AIDS also experience a loss of the sense of time. With AIDS in the family, however, there is no way to put the experience behind. For many children the losses just keep coming. Keeping a calendar, learning about the passage of time, and creating positive temporal benchmarks can be an essential part of the therapeutic work with young children whose parents are sick with AIDS.

> Emma was almost four years old when she entered therapy. An angry and fearful child who was given to nonverbal temper outbursts, she could not express in words her frustration about her life situation with an HIV-infected mother—who was herself mad, sad, and scared. Emma's therapy centered on play, especially with Play-Doh. In each session, she would try to make a birthday cake, and each time she would end up throwing the cake, usually at the therapist. This repetitive behavior was associated with the loss of her father, who had disappeared after celebrating her third birthday with her.
>
> The therapist talked with Emma about birthdays, about being one, two, three, four, and soon five. One day after several months of therapy, Emma made a birthday cake with five distinct candles on it. Over time Emma's fear that her anger had caused her father to leave had abated, and the therapist sensed that this cake would not be smashed—that Emma was ready for a celebration. The therapist no longer needed to duck the flying Play-Doh, and Emma had found herself a birthday and a future, at least until her mother becomes ill.

The Caregivers' Burden

People who work with children of war are often from the same ethnic background as the children. They work in a politically charged atmosphere, but one with camaraderie and mutual support. For therapists working with survivors of war, there are also significant and difficult countertransference problems, especially if the survivors are now in another country, such as rage at the evil of the perpetrators, identification with the victim, and feeling retraumatized by the intensity of reliving the survivor's experience in the retelling.[15] Those who work with children of war have found ways to support each other, to deal with unspeakable trauma through nonverbal means, to pace themselves.

With children surviving AIDS, the work of the caretakers is still in its early stages, and their task is complex. All the stigma and isolation of the children is there for the caregivers as well. Caregivers may feel reluctant to share the pain of their work with loved ones and friends because the telling could reveal the stigmatizing secret of their patients or seem too sad to those who don't know people with AIDS.

Also, like the support system for those who work with children of war, the societal infrastructure for dealing with HIV disease is compromised and overwhelmed. There is the illusion and the hope of social services and supports for everyone, but the systems are inadequate, antiquated, unresponsive. Overwhelmed caretakers bear the sadness and feel the terror and agony of the families they treat. Therapists identify with vulnerability, and the child who is being orphaned by AIDS is very vulnerable. Universal rescue fantasies make therapists want to give back to the children what cannot be replaced. Caregivers also identify with the dying parents. If those parents get angry at the caregivers for surviving, their antagonism may present the children with a loyalty conflict and make the caregivers less physically and emotionally available to the children.

Caretakers who work with AIDS, like the families they help, feel the need for safety, for protection from the assaults, and for some sanctuary. They need to work within the available systems, but at the same time they feel the need to define the specialness of the AIDS situation, a need to gather in others who have relevant experience (with epidemics or orphans, for example) and to build a network of support. Such a supportive network can empower caregivers with esprit de corps and provide a necessary emotional antidote to AIDS. This lesson has been learned by those who work with children of war and is being applied by those who work with all kinds of trauma, including AIDS.

Responding to Children Affected by AIDS

In framing our response to children affected by AIDS, a useful model is our response to children suffering from the trauma and stresses of any disaster.[16] We know that three important factors help children survive such major stresses: (1) the child's temperament; (2) family support—a stable adult in the home or extended family and friends—who can maintain a sense of cohesiveness; and (3) external support.[17] Of the three factors, the first two are the hardest to influence.

The child who engages caregivers, who has modulated activity and good cognitive skills, and who is able to seek and use support is likely to be more resilient to stress. However difficult it is to change temperament, we must encourage and support programs that will best promote these coping mechanisms in children.

We also want to encourage and support families to make individual arrangements for each child, to build connections to cultural roots and supports (church, neighborhood, family), and to use elders and culturally sensitive activities and materials (crafts, music) that keep children connected to their roots and give them a sense of continuity even as deaths have broken the continuity of their lives.

Supporting the children's caregivers, who in turn provide external support for the children, is another way to help these children survive the major stresses in their lives. Support groups, activities that affirm life, diversions from work, and diversification of work are all ways to support caregivers.

The children, too, need other external supports outside the family. We can help them find others who are similarly affected by AIDS, with whom they can "break the silence"; provide group homes (for those children who cannot bear being dependent on a single adult); provide access to therapy with trained clinicians; create and operate school-based programs and curricula that acknowledge the impact of the epidemic and provide settings in which they can maximize their resilient capacities; provide neighborhood drop-in centers; give them opportunities for nonverbal, constructive expressions of despair—such as art projects.

The lessons we have learned about children in war, though still incomplete, can help guide us in our work with children affected by HIV. Both groups of children experience multiple losses and feelings of shame, responsibility, and isolation. For both, the process of emotional rebuilding takes the survivors a lifetime and often extends to future generations.

Children living with HIV, however, face some unique challenges. These child survivors are not so readily incorporated into their communities, and they are further isolated by the stigmatization, shame, and secrecy surrounding this disease. For children who are the survivors of physical wars, the enemy is often identifiable. The enemy may be persons of another race, culture, religion, or ethnicity. Children on either side of this type of war are bonded to their respective communities and are often taken in when orphaned by virtue of their sameness. In contrast, for children who are the survivors of AIDS in their families, the enemy cannot be seen. It is a virus that is embodied by a parent or a sibling. If children were to try to fight and destroy the "enemy," their target would be their parents, siblings, or even themselves.

HIV involves some of the most vulnerable members of our society and results in a devastation as severe as what has been seen in war zones, yet much more subtle. The cost of HIV to children now, and to generations of children after, has just begun. These survivors are *our* children, and until we acknowledge that HIV is not a disease "of others," but one that can infect any one of us, we will continue to add to their pain.

Notes

1. Freud, A., 1946, *The ego and the mechanism of defence,* New York: International Universities Press.

2. This observation is based on interviews conducted by Doctor Apfel and Dr. Bennett Simon with numerous Holocaust survivors between 1989 and 1993.

3. Bar-On, D., 1989, *Legacy of silence: Encounters with children of the Third Reich,* Cambridge: Harvard University Press.

4. Freud, A., and D. Burlingham, 1943, *Children and war,* London: Medical War Books.

5. Bryce, J., 1989, Life experiences, response styles, and mental health among mothers and children in Beirut, Lebanon, *Social Science and Medicine* 28: 685–695.

6. Volkan, V. D., 1990, Living statues and political decision making, *Mind & Human Interaction* (special issue on children in war) 2 (2): 46–50.

7. Konner, M., 1989, Anthropology and psychiatry: Childhood experience and adult predisposition, in *Comprehensive textbook of psychiatry,* 5th ed., ed. H. I. Kaplan and B. J. Sadock, sec. 4, 290–291, Baltimore: Williams and Wilkins; Garmezy, N., 1986, Developmental aspects of children's responses to the stress of separation and loss, in *Depression in young people: Developmental and clinical perspectives,* ed. M. Rutter, C. Izard, and P. Read. New York: Guilford.

8. Nemiah, J., 1961, Pathological grief, in *Foundations of psychopathology,* New York: Oxford University Press, 168–197.

9. For discussion of the child survivors of World War II, see D. Dwork, 1991, *Children with a star: Jewish youth in Nazi Europe,* New Haven: Yale University Press; Moskovitz, S., 1983, *Love despite hate: Child survivors of the Holocaust and their adult lives,* New York: Schocken.

10. Macksoud, M. S., 1993, *Helping children cope with the stresses of war: A manual for parents and teachers.* New York: UNICEF.

11. See Resource Guide for information about obtaining *My personal life history: A guided activity workbook for foster children, their families, caseworkers, and teachers.* Dr. Kliman is the founder of the Foster Care Study Unit, Department of Child Psychiatry, Columbia University College of Physicians and Surgeons.

12. Yassen, J., Workshops on secondary traumatization, Cambridge Hospital Victims of Violence program, personal communication.

13. Moskovitz, see note 9 above.

14. Durban, J., and P. Palgi, 1993, chapter 25, The role and function of collective representations for the individual during the mourning process: The case of a war bereaved boy (Hebrew with English summary), in *Loss and bereavement in Jewish society in Israel,* ed. R. Malkinson, S. Rubin, and E. Witztum, Jerusalem: Cana.

15. Herman, J. L., 1992, *Trauma and recovery,* New York: Basic.

16. Galante, R., and D. Foa, 1986, An epidemiological study of psychic trauma and treatment effectiveness for children after a natural disaster, *Journal of the American Academy of Child Psychiatry* 25: 357–363.

17. Garmezy, N., 1985, Stress-resistant children: The search for protective factors, *Journal of Child Psychology and Psychiatry Supplement* 4: 213–233.

Part Three

Responding to the Needs of Children and Youth Affected by AIDS

Chapter 8

A Second Family?
Placement and Custody Decisions
BARBARA DRAIMIN

Maria is a thirty-six-year-old Puerto Rican mother with AIDS who has three children, ages fourteen, eight and six. The eldest child's father is deceased. The father of the eight- and six-year-old does not live with the family and sees the children only once or twice a year. Maria insisted that he leave their apartment four years ago after he came home drunk and hit her and the children. He provides no financial or emotional support and knows nothing about the HIV disease within the family.

Maria has a large extended family, including a sister and her four children, and a divorced brother. Maria's mother is sixty years old. She is emotionally close to the children and lives in the same building, but she is handicapped by severe arthritis. Maria has told her sister and her fourteen-year-old son about having AIDS, but she has not told her mother, brother, or her two younger children. There is no custody plan. She does not want her three children to be separated, but she fears that no one can take all three of them. Although the eldest child helps care for her and for the younger children, he cannot become the substitute parent when Maria dies.

Maria prays that the family will "figure out something" because they have always pulled together in the past. A hospital social worker suggested that they begin a formal custody planning process, but Maria knows that her extended family would be insulted by such a procedure. Taking responsibility for "family" is not a matter that should involve lawyers or any other outsiders; she believes it is simply the duty of family members to come forward and care for one another.

As we have seen in other chapters, parents with HIV disease who have uninfected children reflect increasing diversity in family heritage, economic circumstance, and geographic location. Regardless of background, all of these parents have difficult issues to address: their own anger, depression, and sadness over the illness; the reality of their impending death; the need to keep family secrets about the nature of their illness; and the response of their children to their progressive incapacity to care for themselves and their families. Perhaps the most difficult task they face, however, is the need to make a choice regarding the future placement and custody of their children. Like Maria, many of these parents—most often women—have difficulty beginning the planning process, in part because of cultural expectations about the obligations of family or because of negative experiences with such "helping agents" as social workers, lawyers, and welfare or other government agencies. Some infected parents have difficulty navigating the often confusing web of legal options and social services that might assist them in their search for a second family for their children. Still others cannot successfully consummate the process of "handing over" their parental relationship with their children to another family.

This chapter discusses a range of issues that arise when HIV-infected parents plan for a new placement and new guardians for their children. It describes myths and realities about what parents want and what actually occurs; it explains how the social, legal, and entitlement systems may both hinder and assist a parent's ability to plan for her children; and it identifies supports that can improve the chances of a successful custody change for the child and the new family. Finally, it replaces myths with facts essential to improved clinical understanding and policy planning on behalf of these children.

Myths and Data

Myth: Most AIDS orphans end up living in foster care.

Myth: Most times, siblings will be able to continue to live together in a new family.

Myth: The eldest teen often becomes the legal guardian for his or her younger siblings.

Myth: Mothers with AIDS usually do not make custody plans because they are in denial about their own illness.

Myth: A parent cannot successfully effect a custody plan until she has disclosed her HIV status to her children.

In addressing the realities of custody planning and outcomes for children who have been or will become orphaned by AIDS, we acknowledge the paucity of longitudinal and national research on what happens to these children. We draw our data for this chapter from four recent studies, three having been completed and reported from 1992 to 1994 and one still in progress.

"Biologic, Foster, and Adoptive Parents: Care Givers of Children Exposed Perinatally to Human Immunodeficiency Virus in the United States" (1992)

A report from the Pediatric Spectrum of Disease project by M. Black Caldwell et al., published in *Pediatrics* in 1992, documented the current living situations of 1,683 children born to mothers infected by HIV at six sites (Los Angeles, New York City, Houston/Dallas/San Antonio, Massachusetts, Washington, D.C., and San Francisco).[1] Overall, 56 percent were living with a biologic parent, 10 percent were living with another relative, 27 percent were in foster care, 3 percent had been adopted, and 4 percent were living in group settings or with other caregivers. This distribution did not vary significantly for children whose mothers had died. The distribution did vary by geographic location, however: a greater proportion of exposed children lived with a biologic parent in Texas (70 percent) than in New York City (42 percent); and a greater proportion of children lived in foster care in New York City (41 percent) than in Washington, D.C. (8 percent). The distribution also differed by race/ethnicity: 63 percent of white children and 64 percent of Hispanic children lived with a biologic parent, as compared with 50 percent of African-American children. However, maternal drug use also differed by race/ethnicity, and children born to mothers with HIV who used intravenous drugs were more likely to have been living with alternative caregivers.

"The Mental Health Needs of Well Adolescents in Families with AIDS" (1992)

The second study, completed in September 1991 by the New York City Human Resources Administration Division of AIDS Services (DAS), assessed the mental health needs of well adolescents aged ten to nineteen living in families with AIDS.[2] The design and findings of this study are discussed fully in Chapter 5. Of note here are its findings pertaining to disclosure and custody planning. The interviews with parents and new guardians in this study documented the family's difficulties with these issues. In 53 percent of the families where the parent was alive, there was no viable custody plan for the adolescent children. A plan was defined as *viable* if it was proposed by the parent and agreed upon by the adolescent and the new guardian. It was not unusual in these families for a relative to agree to be the guardian for the younger children but to refuse responsibility for the adolescent—particularly for an adolescent who was "acting out." In 10 percent of the families, older adolescents assumed guardianship of their young siblings in order to keep all the children together.

"In Whose Care and Custody" (1993)

The third study, completed by the DAS in conjunction with The Orphan Project in New York City, assessed where children were living twelve months after a parent's death from AIDS.[3] The study further examined the effect of financial support, access to suitable and affordable housing, and emotional support services on the permanency of these children's placements. The sample consisted of forty-three families with 108 children, or the caseload of one DAS case manager. Demographic characteristics of these families reflected the DAS caseload: 40 percent of the families were African-American, 51 percent Hispanic, and 9 percent Anglo-American. Seventy-four percent of the parents with AIDS were female.

For 33 percent of these cases, no custody plan had been made for the children, and for an additional 12 percent the custody planning process was not documentable, the family having moved out of state or refused services from DAS. Of the twenty-four families with custody plans, only eight had utilized the assistance of legal services in drawing up documents formally naming the selected person as the new guardian, and none had gone to family court to formally confirm the new guardians by the time the case was closed by DAS, shortly after the parent's death. In the remaining sixteen cases, a new guardian had been named by the parent, but no steps had been taken to formalize this selection.

Of the twenty-four cases with custody plans, grandparents and aunts functioned as the new guardians in fourteen, a family friend in three, and the other biological parent in four. An older sibling, a kinship foster parent, and a godparent became the new guardians in the remaining three cases. Across all cases, those with plans and those without, siblings remained together only 43 percent of the time, and the New York City Child Welfare Administration was involved in 14 percent of these cases.

"Interventions for Adolescents Whose Parents Live with AIDS" (Ongoing)

The final study, also funded by the National Institute of Mental Health, is currently under way under the aegis of the University of California at Los Angeles and the DAS in New York City.[4] This prospective, randomized intervention study is following the adolescents aged twelve to eighteen of 360 mothers with AIDS, newly registered with DAS, to study the efficacy of various strategies designed to enhance coping skills and thereby reduce the negative outcomes for these adolescents. Assessments at three-month intervals over a twenty-four-month period examine adolescents' outcomes (mental health, behavior, social adjustment), factors mediating adjustment, and background factors. Through this study, it will be possible to report more definitively on how often the placement of the child matched the plan intended by the parent and how permanent these placements were for the children in them. Participants in the study reflect the general DAS caseload; 53 percent are African-American, 40 percent are Hispanic, and 7 percent are Anglo-American.

Data relevant to this chapter are drawn from baseline information on parents' plans for their children gathered during the pilot stage and the initial enrollment of study subjects. Preliminary data on parental plans involving thirty families and fifty-nine children show that only seven of the thirty families had made a formal custody plan involving legal documents. Of the remaining twenty-three families, only four had an informal plan about which both the child and potential guardian knew and to which they agreed. The other nineteen families had either thought about a possible guardian but had not informed this person or had made no plans at all for their children's future. When parents were asked whom they expected to take care of their children, guardianship usually fell to the immediate family members of the parent with AIDS: 53 percent of the children were expected to stay with grandparents, aunts, and uncles, 20 percent with the surviving parent, and 8 percent with older siblings. Fourteen percent of the children were to be placed with non-relatives and 5 percent with godparents. Most of the parents' plans failed to address important contingency issues for their children and new guardians, such as housing, financial support, age and health of the new guardian, and connection with the extended family. For example, 73 percent of the parents expected that all of their children would remain together, regardless of the number of children in the family. The chance that this will happen is very slim, based on field observations of caseworkers in New York City.

The Studies in Sum

Taken together, these four studies begin to call into question several of the myths identified at the beginning of this chapter. First, even in the absence of formal custody planning by many parents, the vast majority of the AIDS "orphans" go to live with family members, at least in the first year after the death of the parent. Additional research that tracks these children over longer periods of time is needed to understand and help plan for placements that accord with parental wishes and meet the psychosocial needs of the children. We also need to understand whether family members, especially grandparents, are able to maintain these new caregiving responsibilities over an extended period of time.

Second, although the parent with AIDS hopes and intends that her children remain together, that appears to occur less than half of the time; adolescents are particularly difficult to place with other siblings.

Issues in the Custody Planning Process

Talking about Illness in the Family

As reported in other chapters and in the prospective, ongoing NIMH study described earlier in this chapter, many adults find it exceedingly difficult to talk about having HIV disease with their children, their own parents, and others. One factor contributing to this difficulty may be the word some professionals use to describe the act of telling: *disclosure*. The word may well convey a negative value judgment to the parent. To disclose is to *confess, divulge, reveal, bare,* or *uncover*. The word itself may contribute to the stigma of AIDS; as professionals, we need to change our use of it. We need to explore with family members how they communicate about important things in one another's lives. How do they share successes and losses? Talking about HIV must be done within the context of how family members listen and speak to one another.

Parents and professionals sometimes believe that talking about HIV disease is an all-or-nothing process. Afraid of what their children or others will ask, infected parents may prefer to say nothing until the virus results in debilitating illness. Parents may see *naming* and *telling* as a slippery slope that begins with a discussion of the illness but ends with the question, "How did you get AIDS?" Many parents need professional help to understand that they can talk about the disease in more general terms and over a period of time, during which they control and direct the amount and nature of information provided to the child or children.

An alternative to parents' naming their present or future illness specifically as HIV or AIDS is to begin talking about their health using only the term *illness*. Opportunities to talk about illness in the family may include: (*a*) the time of the parent's diagnosis; (*b*) the HIV-related illness of another family member; (*c*) the period during which AZT or other AIDS-identified medications are present in the home; (*d*) the time when the parent begins to experience HIV-associated illnesses; (*e*) the time when the parent needs hospitalization, respite care, or homemaker services in the home; (*f*) the onset of progressively terminal illness. The presence of a trusted professional or member of the clergy can enable the parent to begin the process of *telling* in a way appropriate to the stage of the disease and to the developmental capacity of the child or children.

In some instances, having brought the helping professional to the discussion with the children, the parent will be unable to verbalize or even participate in the intended discussion, and the professional will be called upon to make a judgment about whether to speak for the parent, and what to say. Most professionals will choose not to speak for the parent, but to reschedule at a subsequent time. The professional or some other trusted adult must be available to the child as a source of support in processing and coping with the information given. Affected children who do not receive support at this point may engage in extreme withdrawal or acting out behaviors as they attempt to respond to the situation.[5]

The act of *not talking* about one's HIV disease may actually serve an important therapeutic function for an adult, as denial functions to keep the individual looking ahead toward a hopeful future. But for the parent with children, the inability to talk about the disease can lead the children to create their own hypotheses about what they actually see happening to the parent. Too often, the child will conclude that his or her own behavior is the cause of the illness. In addition, children begin to form unspoken questions about who will take care of them if something happens to the parent.

V. N. Niebuhr et al. recently found that 90 percent of the white, 60 percent of the Hispanic, and 56 percent of the African-American parents in their survey in Texas reported that their children knew of their diagnosis of HIV.[6] Significantly more data are required before we fully understand how and when children are told or come to understand about HIV in their families, and what role culture plays in the decision to reveal or conceal the diagnosis.

Beginning the Process of Custody Planning

Parents are dealing with the issue of whether, when, and how to talk with their children about illness at the same time that they confront the need to make a plan. It is limiting for professionals and clients to believe that concerns about talking about the illness must be resolved before the task of custody planning can begin. Custody planning is an emotionally complex process often made even more difficult by confusing and sometimes contradictory legal and social service regulations, and by the incapacitating effects of the disease.

Other factors may also inhibit a parent's ability to plan for a change in custody. Like Maria, the parent may be bound by cultural tradition to anticipate that one or more extended family members will step in at the point of her death and take her children to their home. Or, having talked with the child about her illness, the parent may fear hurting the child further with talk about death and the need to move in with a new family. Some parents who have several children, including an adolescent, may believe that the adolescent is capable of becoming the emotional and legal surrogate parent to the younger siblings. Such plans for adolescent guardianship need special attention. A parent who views adolescent guardianship as the only way to keep the siblings together may be placing unrealistic demands on the young person. In group sessions with adolescents, these youths have discussed parental pressure and their own guilt as motivating factors that lead them to accept more responsibility than they know is possible to fulfill. Co-guardianship with an adult may provide one alternative that affords significant support to the adolescent. Parents whose children have engaged in increasingly antisocial, destructive, or dangerous behaviors may believe that no placement options are available for the child. Clearly, there is more involved in a parent's inability to begin the process of custody planning than denial of her own condition.

As professionals, we can predict that HIV-infected parents will wrestle with some or all of the following questions in the custody-planning process:

- Can I keep my children together?
- What special medical or psychological needs does each have?
- What should I do about my surviving spouse, whom I may not want to contact?
- Of the people I know, whom do I trust the most to care for my children?
- How do I begin to talk with the prospective guardian about custody?
- Do I have to tell a new guardian about my illness? How much? When?
- Should a new guardian begin taking care of the children now?
- Is the new guardian healthy, and does he or she have the space to care for all of my children?
- Do the children need money and other resources?
- What happens if I don't make a plan?
- Will my family find some way to work it out?
- What do my children want?

These intimate and complicated questions may first be expressed in the context of discussions with a trusted medical adviser, a close friend or family member, or a member of the clergy. However, ideally, each parent who begins to explore custody options for her children would have the help of a multi-disciplinary team, including at least a mental health professional, an attorney, and an entitlement specialist, all of whom are trained in family therapy, child development, custody law, and the HIV disease process. Ideally the infected parent would begin to work on custody issues no later than six months to a year before being incapacitated by illness. In reality, however, a parent infected by HIV cannot predict with any certainty how long she will remain healthy and, once her immune system becomes severely compromised, how soon she will die. In addition, any infected parent would be fortunate to find an attorney, a social worker, or entitlement specialist who is fully knowledgeable in the range and requirements of custody options and consequences of various choices.

Professionals who assist parents in a custody planning process must be sensitive to timing and pacing. Frequently the professional, understanding how long the legal and financial processes on behalf of the child can take, sees the need to move quickly because of the deteriorating health of the parent. There is a danger, however, in assertive prodding on the part of the professional. As noted in the mental health assessment study, when parents present too much information about their illness and inevitable death and when there is inadequate mental health support for their children, both children and adolescents may respond with attempts to take their own lives.[7]

Even early and complete custody planning cannot negate all hazards. Joint parenting, with the parents and designated caretakers working closely together in the care of the child, can raise difficult issues of loyalty and allegiance. In one case we are following in the Division of AIDS Services, an elementary school child awoke one morning and tiptoed into his mother's room to get his report card signed. Her breathing was shallow and she was sweating profusely. The child summoned the health aide and decided not to wake his mother to sign his report card. Instead, he went to his prospective guardian's house and asked her to sign it. Four days later, his mother asked what had happened to his report card. She became very angry at the child, and at the new guardian for usurping her parental role. Another parent whose children were being cared for by both herself and a new guardian said, "I thought everyone was waiting for me to die. Even though they tried to let me be head of the family, I became so weak and sick that I could not remember things. Naturally, the children started depending on their new guardians. It almost killed me. I was glad to have help but greatly resented that they would see my children graduate and I would not." With professional counseling, the families in both examples were able to work through their ambivalence, but these incidents speak eloquently to the difficulty that the ill parent may have in handing over parental responsibility to another family.

Legal Options for Transferring Custody

Formalization of a parent's wishes for the guardianship of children may take many months and requires the early assistance of a lawyer skilled in custody matters. The legal options available to a parent with a terminal disease may vary from state to state, but typically include (a) development of a will that names the parent's choice of new guardian but requires judicial approval of the choice after the parent's death; (b) designation of legal guardian before the death of the parent (and, in a few states, designation of a stand-by guardian); (c) termination of the parent's legal rights and adoption by another adult; or (d) entry of the child into the child welfare foster care system. These options are discussed in detail in Chapter 9.

Financial Supports

One of the major issues facing the parent infected by HIV, as well as the new guardian, involves continued eligibility of the child and the new family for financial support. Regulations concerning eligibility may vary by municipality, state, and governing agency, and they can be difficult for a parent or family to obtain and understand. Some entitlements are calculated based on the individual budgets of each family, making it virtually impossible for anyone outside the welfare system to calculate what a family might be eligible to receive. When a family is entitled to financial aid from more than one agency, regulations may be contradictory, and because information sharing is notoriously difficult, the task of traversing a web of cross-agency regulations may seem impossible.

A child who moves from a specialized AIDS caseload to the more general caseloads of the public assistance agency, usually upon the death of the parent, has much less opportunity to obtain individualized attention. In New York City the specialized AIDS caseloads are thirty-six families or individuals per worker; entitlement workers serving public welfare cases carry a caseload of 190 families. Also, when a child or family moves from AIDS-specific services, service and benefits are often interrupted.

The following simplified listing identifies entitlements for children that are most often misunderstood by parents and new guardians. These programs are based on the needs of the child and do not relate to the income of the new guardian, though the new guardian's income and taxes may be affected by the children's entitlements.

Aid to Families with Dependent Children (AFDC). In the AFDC program, when a caretaker relative—someone within a degree of kinship specified in federal law—assumes care of children, that relative is eligible to receive AFDC benefits on behalf of the children. The caretaker relative may be required to show proof of the death of the parent but does not have to secure legal guardianship status in order to receive aid. The caretaker relative can apply for and accept AFDC payments without reporting his or her income level. Food stamp applications, by contrast, require income information from all household members. Guardians who do not wish to provide income information can choose to forgo food stamp entitlements and yet still receive AFDC benefits.

Foster Care Assistance. Foster care rates are provided to those licensed by the state child welfare agency. These rates are more generous than AFDC, particularly when two or more children are in the home. In New York a licensed foster parent with three children is eligible for $1,350 per month from foster care, compared with $552 monthly from AFDC. AFDC rates vary widely among states, but on average are 50 percent lower than foster care rates.[8] Relatives who become licensed foster parents to children eligible for Title IV-E foster care payments are entitled to full foster care rates, though not all states in fact pay them these rates. Unfortunately, if a parent has a relative appointed a guardian/stand-by guardian, that relative will be disqualified from future kinship foster care benefits, penalizing the new guardian (especially a grandparent) for years to come. Foster care also means that the commissioner of the child welfare agency is the child's legal guardian and that the agency has monitoring and oversight responsibilities of the foster family and the child.

Social Security Benefits. Social security provides two types of benefits for eligible children. If the parent worked, paid social security taxes, and earned enough credits, surviving children are eligible for Social Security Survivor benefits if they are unmarried and under age eighteen (nineteen if attending elementary or secondary school full time, or up to age twenty-one if attending college). To receive Supplemental Security Income (SSI), the surviving child must be blind or disabled.

Federal Adoption Assistance. Children who are eligible for federally funded foster care may also be eligible for adoption assistance if they have special needs or are hard to place. Rates vary by state.

The Needs of New Guardians

In addition to the need for financial supports, the new guardians of children orphaned by AIDS face a number of challenges. New guardians who are relatives of the deceased parent have the dual task of dealing with the loss of their own loved one at the same time they are helping the surviving children through their own bereavement process. Both the new guardian and the surviving children are concurrently dealing with change and loss. The transition in households, in schools, and in reconstituted families makes a quiet and supportive mourning period unlikely. At a time when children need consistent support and understanding, they are more likely to encounter chaos and enormous change. Children whose families kept AIDS a secret from them may feel that they lack permission to have and share feelings about the life and death of the parent. These children may not be able to mourn until they have engaged in significant acting out behaviors.

Housing presents another challenge to new guardians who are relatives of the deceased parent with AIDS. When the new guardian is an aunt within the family, she often still has children of her own in a fully occupied apartment or home, with little room to absorb two or three additional children. Grandparents who become guardians may live in a small apartment that suited them well after their children moved out but has little room for several children. Even if the grandparents are willing to move into the children's present home, there may be a restriction against it. If the family occupied housing through a specialized rental assistance program for persons with AIDS or lived in an AIDS-dedicated housing unit, for example, neither the surviving children nor the new guardian will qualify to keep that housing.

All new guardians also face the enormous and complicated task of helping the children become integrated into the guardian's existing family with all of its rules and expectations. Older children who have taken on a parental role for their siblings during the illness of their parent often find it difficult to return to the role of subservient child, taking rather than giving orders. In the sadness and chaos of terminal illness, family discipline may have lapsed, and children may have become accustomed to missing school and having no structured times for eating and sleeping. This conflict may be even more intense when the new guardian is a grandparent who remembers parenting according to behaviors and expectations of a generation ago. Because customs and generational norms have changed over time, both children and grandparents will have to modify their expectations about roles and behavior.

Finally, as discussed earlier, when the new guardian is an adolescent sibling, this additional responsibility puts enormous pressure on both the younger siblings and the adolescent. Sharing parenting responsibilities between the adolescent and another adult offers the best likelihood of success.

Service Models

Communities struggling with AIDS and these difficult issues have developed models for service to help ease this painful transition. New York City, a community working with these problems for well over a decade, provides six models (addresses and telephone numbers are included in the Resource Guide):

Early Permanency Planning

Early Permanency Planning (EPP) was implemented in 1992 by the New York City Child Welfare Administration to help parents with terminal illness use the foster care system in a voluntary and friendly manner. Designed for parents who have not designated an individual to assume legal guardianship of their children, EPP is designed to prevent emergency placements of the children at the time of the parents' deaths. At the parents' request, the child welfare agency helps identify a home with a relative, friend, or stranger. The designated caretaker is specifically prepared to care for the children through the establishment of a permanent preadoptive home. The parent signs a voluntary placement agreement so the children can enter care when the parent believes placement is necessary. Parents are referred to legal services for help in preparing documents. Supportive services are provided to build a trusting relationship between the biologic and foster families.

Family Crisis Treatment

The Well Children in AIDS Families Project, run by Beth Israel Medical Center, began providing mental health services to well children in families with AIDS in 1987. The original support group model was changed to a family crisis treatment model. Parents are offered consultations to help them talk about AIDS, and the program provides ongoing counseling to children. If a custody dispute between maternal and paternal sides of the family seems possible, a family meeting is convened to mediate the dispute before a court becomes involved.

Transitional Case Management

The Family Center for Services and Research provides transitional service to parents, children, and the new guardians. Started in 1994, and one of the first of its kind, the program specializes in walking parents through the issues of planning for their children's futures, including talking about AIDS and custody planning. A highly trained case management staff is supplemented by a team that consists of a social worker, an attorney, and an entitlement specialist, who assess each case through weekly case conferences.

Parent and Adolescent Groups

The NIMH-funded prospective intervention study discussed earlier provides a range of services to the 180 families in the experimental group.[9] Started in March 1993, it is designed to measure the impact of a program that seeks to enhance the coping skills of well adolescents. The program provides a sixteen-day intervention that involves parent groups, youth groups, and combined groups. The curriculum includes sessions on coping with illness, telling others, custody planning, and parent-child communication. The three sessions with parents and youths together focus on creating a positive atmosphere at home, resolving conflicts, and working together on custody plans.

Three-Generational Intervention

The Community Consultation Center at the Henry Street Settlement House has developed a three-generation intervention model that seeks to repair the relationship between the mother with AIDS and her own parents and birth family to help ensure success for placements of her children with extended family members after her death. Henry Street provides individual, group, and family bereavement counseling, and runs school-based bereavement groups for healthy children affected by AIDS deaths in their families.

Child Psychiatric Services

The Special Needs Clinic at Columbia-Presbyterian Medical Center provides HIV-focused child psychiatric services to children from families living with AIDS. Rather than responding to crises occurring after a parent's death, clinical social workers on the staff try to identify children who are at risk for mental health problems or are already demonstrating them in response to parental HIV-related illness. The clinic stresses individual therapy for these children (two-thirds of whom are not infected) as well as family therapy. It actively engages in research efforts to assess the impact of HIV on these children and the effectiveness of various mental health interventions with them.

We must work to improve legal, mental health, and entitlement systems at the same time as we acknowledge the limitations of systems to serve the unique and resilient nature of each family.

As professionals, we are humbled by the enormity of each family's challenges, and the courage needed to face them. *Our* challenge is to create programs that will support all family members, and to change our often irrational systems. Additional research will expand our knowledge base and reduce the myths that interfere with our progress.

> *Fact:* Most AIDS orphans go to live with family members, especially aunts and grandmothers. Most do *not* end up in foster care or with the eldest teenage sibling as guardian.
>
> *Fact:* Siblings are often separated because it is hard for the future guardian to take in more than two children, or because child welfare regulations in some states may limit the number of children who may be placed in a foster home.
>
> *Fact:* Parents do not make placement plans because there is no one they trust to take care of their children. Denial about their illness can be a factor, but is not the overwhelming one.
>
> *Fact:* Acknowledging illness is important to custody planning. HIV disclosure is *not* a prerequisite to starting a custody plan.

Notes

1. Caldwell, M. B., et al., 1992, Biologic, foster, and adoptive parents: Care givers of children exposed perinatally to human immunodeficiency virus in the United States, *Pediatrics* 90: 603–607.

2. Draimin, B., J. Hudis, and J. Segura, 1992, *The mental health needs of well adolescents in families with AIDS,* New York: New York City Human Resources Administration, Division of AIDS Services.

3. Gamble, I., 1993, *In whose care and custody,* New York: New York City Human Resources Administration, Division of AIDS Services.

4. Rotheram-Borus, M. J., and B. Draimin, 1992, *Interventions for adolescents whose parents live with AIDS,* NIMH Grant MH49958-03.

5. Draimin et al., see note 2 above.

6. Niebuhr, V. N., J. R. Hughes, and R. B. Pollard, 1994, Parents with human immunodeficiency virus infection: Perceptions of their children's emotional needs, *Pediatrics* 93: 421–426. See also K. Siegel and E. Gorey, 1994, Childhood bereavement due to parental death from acquired immunodeficiency syndrome, *Journal of Developmental and Behavioral Pediatrics* 15 (3): S66–S70 (June supplement); the authors discuss the particular importance of secrecy for many minority families.

7. Draimin et al., see note 2 above.

8. United States House of Representatives Committee on Ways and Means, 1993, *Overview of entitlement programs: 1993 Green Book,* Washington, D.C.: Government Printing Office.

9. Additional information about this study can be obtained through the principal investigators, Mary J. Rotheram-Borus, University of California at Los Angeles, and Barbara Draimin, New York City Human Resources Administration, Division of AIDS Services, 212-966-8168.

Chapter 9

Toward a Child-Responsive Legal System

SHELLEY GEBALLE

The law can neither cure AIDS nor prevent its spread. The law can, however, be more responsive to children facing AIDS in their families. This chapter discusses three targets for improvement: (*a*) combating the stigma that surrounds AIDS; (*b*) reducing the trauma associated with changes in custody; and (*c*) protecting the health of the surviving children. Each section first summarizes existing law and its limitations, then recommends necessary changes. In painting this picture of how the law might improve its responsiveness, the chapter uses the broadest of brush strokes, leaving detail to others.

Combating AIDS Stigma

More than a decade into the pandemic, AIDS still carries enormous stigma that traps families in silence and, in turn, limits their ability to gain support from others and to plan for the future. HIV-related discrimination also continues, harming not only persons who are infected but also persons *perceived* to be infected, as well as uninfected family members and caregivers. The law targets this stigma by providing people affected by HIV with some recourse against illegal discrimination and by giving them some control over who gains access to HIV-related information.

Protection Against Discrimination

Recent changes in federal and state law have expanded markedly the protection against HIV-related discrimination. Three federal statutes provide children from families with HIV disease significant recourse against discriminatory conduct: the Americans with Disabilities Act (the ADA), Section 504 of the Rehabilitation Act of 1973, and the Fair Housing Act Amendments of 1988 (the FHAA).

The ADA, enacted in July 1990, protects against discrimination in employment, public accommodations, transportation, and public services. Persons with disability or with a record of disability, as well as nondisabled persons who are regarded as having a disability, are protected by the ADA. The ADA draws substantively from the Rehabilitation Act (which bars discrimination by federally funded and operated programs against otherwise qualified individuals with handicaps) and procedurally from Title VII of the Civil Rights Act of 1964 (in its remedies and remedial process). Decisions interpreting the Rehabilitation Act and the ADA, as well as their legislative histories, have established that persons with, or perceived as having, HIV disease are considered "disabled" and entitled to protection.

The ADA expands the protection against discrimination in one way which is particularly helpful to well children from families with HIV disease and their caregivers. The ADA expressly prohibits discrimination in employment and in public accommodations against any person based on that person's relationship or association with a person with a disability. Children and other family members, caregivers, friends, neighbors, advocates, employees and volunteers of social service agencies, and foster and adoptive parents all fall within this broadened zone of protection.

The ADA covers all aspects of employment (job application procedures and hiring decisions, for example, as well as compensation, fringe benefits, job assignments, and firing). An employer cannot refuse to hire a person because his or her dependents have health conditions that might prove costly to the employer, nor can he fire someone for working with an AIDS services group, for example. The ADA also prohibits discrimination by places of "public accommodation," broadly defined to include more than five million private establishments, including social service agencies (homeless shelters and adoption agencies, for example), hotels and restaurants, stores, schools, and service establishments (doctors' offices, hospitals, travel agencies, for example). A day care center that denied admission to a child because the child's sibling had AIDS, for example, would be violating the ADA.

Those who prove employment discrimination under the ADA can receive job reinstatement, injunctive relief, back pay, compensatory damages (for emotional pain, for example) if the discrimination was intentional, and punitive damages in cases of malice or reckless indifference to rights. Those who prove discrimination by places of public accommodation under the ADA can secure injunctive relief; in suits brought by the attorney general, money damages and civil penalties as high as $100,000 also may be awarded.

The FHAA bars discrimination in the sale or rental of most housing, as well as the use of exclusionary zoning regulations to restrict access to housing. Like the ADA, it protects not only persons with disabilities but also persons who associate with persons with disabilities, including HIV infection. It also bars discrimination based on race or color, national origin, sex, religion and "familial status." Familial status discrimination, as defined broadly in the FHAA, embraces families in which one or more children under age eighteen lives with either a parent, a person who has legal custody of the child, or the designees of the parent or legal custodian. The FHAA has been used successfully to invalidate local zoning restrictions on homes for persons with AIDS and their families and to challenge citizen use of local zoning law to exclude foster homes from residential single-family areas. Foster parents have successfully used the FHAA to challenge other types of housing discrimination against their families. The FHAA also makes it unlawful to coerce, intimidate, threaten, or interfere with any person in the exercise of any right under the Act. The FHAA's remedy for discrimination can include injunctive relief and actual and punitive damages. Under both the FHAA and the ADA, persons who prove discrimination can recover their attorneys' fees and costs.

State and local laws also may provide protection. All states have enacted antidiscrimination protections for persons with disabilities, and a majority have interpreted disabilities to include HIV disease.[1] More than half of the states that include HIV disease as a disability explicitly forbid discrimination against persons who are *perceived* to be HIV infected, like the child of someone who is infected.[2] In some cases, state law may cover situations not covered by the ADA or FHAA and may provide stronger remedies.

Though substantial, all of these legal protections have limits. The law requires a person to have suffered the harmful effects of discrimination before a court will act. Litigation takes time and money, causes enormous stress, and often results in undesired disclosures of information about the litigants. For some acts of discrimination, the law may provide no remedy or an incomplete one. The ADA, for example, does not protect against employment discrimination if the employer has fewer than fifteen employees. Many state laws offer far more limited protection than the ADA and the FHAA and can require lengthy administrative processes for complaint resolution.

Necessary Changes

To combat the stigma that continues to surround AIDS:

• Federal and state law should be amended as necessary to ensure: (*a*) protection for all persons (including those who are perceived to be disabled and those who associate with a person who is disabled) against HIV-related discrimination from any source; (*b*) prompt resolution of discrimination complaints in a manner that protects litigants' privacy (prompt administrative

review, a private right of action, the ability to file complaints using fictitious names, protective orders to prevent disclosure of HIV-related information); (c) full relief to those who prove discrimination, including compensatory and punitive damages and attorneys' fees and costs.
• Discrimination law must be more effectively enforced: (a) through more aggressive investigations and litigation by human and civil rights agencies, relieving families affected by AIDS of some of these burdens of litigation; (b) by publicizing large damage awards and fines to deter discriminatory conduct by others against persons associated with AIDS, including the surviving children and their new families.

Even with these changes, however, the law cannot end discrimination. It cannot compel people to shed their prejudicial attitudes; our civil rights laws hardly erased racism in this country. Discriminatory attitudes must be challenged in other ways as well. Unfounded fears about transmission of HIV can be calmed by continuing public AIDS education, which communicates accurate information about the modes of transmission and encourages compassion for families living with HIV disease. The strongest challenge to discriminatory attitudes, however, will likely result from HIV's relentless march across all of our geographic and socioeconomic boundaries, ensuring that, in time, AIDS will touch each of our lives in a personal way that leaves little room for judgmental attitudes.

Protections for Privacy

So long as HIV-related discrimination remains pervasive, control over who has knowledge about one's infection remains essential. Though a right of privacy is mentioned explicitly neither in the United States Constitution nor in most state constitutions, courts have held consistently that such a constitutional right exists and that it includes the right to decide when to release medical information about oneself to others. This right is not absolute, however. Although courts agree that the right to privacy encompasses decisions about revealing HIV-related information, they have differed when asked to decide what circumstances justify a nonconsensual disclosure of such information.

More than two-thirds of all states also have enacted HIV-specific confidentiality statutes. In general, they prohibit the disclosure of HIV-related information without the consent of the patient or the patient's authorized representative but allow nonconsensual disclosures in certain limited circumstances, most commonly to: (a) health care personnel providing treatment to the patient; (b) health departments for disease surveillance and partner notification purposes; and (c) persons who have a significant exposure to a patient's blood. Subject to some conditions, a few states (Arizona, Connecticut, and Virginia, for example) permit nonconsensual disclosure of HIV-related information to health providers and facilities when necessary to provide appropriate health care to the child of a patient. Some statutes require notification to certain individuals, such as funeral directors and rape victims. A very few states mandate or allow nonconsensual disclosures to school authorities.[3]

Most states with HIV-specific confidentiality statutes impose civil or criminal sanctions on unlawful disclosures. Civil penalties may be payable to the person whose record was unlawfully disclosed. Criminal sanctions can include fines and/or imprisonment. An increasing number of states forbid redisclosures of confidential HIV-related information to others.

For the well child living in a family with HIV disease, these confidentiality statutes are a mixed blessing. On the one hand, they empower infected family members, giving them more control over who will learn about their illness and, by this selective disclosure, probably reducing the amount of discrimination to which a child is exposed. On the other hand, the mere existence of these separate laws reinforces the stigma surrounding AIDS by perpetuating the view that it is different from other chronic and terminal illnesses. The laws also limit information routinely available to such caregivers of the uninfected children and youths as their teachers, health care providers, and extended family members. Knowledge that a child is witnessing the HIV-related illness and death of parents and siblings may be of great relevance to others caring for the child, but this knowledge may be available only if and when the infected family member chooses to share it. In a state that prohibits redisclosures of HIV-related information, a schoolteacher informed by a student's mother that the mother has HIV disease may not relay this information to the student's teacher for the next year unless the mother is willing—and still able—to consent. As a practical matter, many professionals resort to talking in code, speaking of a parent's "chronic and life-threatening illness" but avoiding the terms "AIDS" or "HIV disease."

Necessary Changes

If and when HIV-related discrimination abates, the continued need for expansive, specific protection for the confidentiality of HIV-related information should be reevaluated. Until that time, however, all protections should remain intact, with one possible exception: allowing limited nonconsensual disclosures among professionals who are providing care to a child when specific knowledge about a parent's HIV-related illness is essential to maintaining that child's physical and mental well-being.

Ensuring Continuity in Placement and Custody

Until AIDS can be cured or more successfully managed as a chronic disease, many children with AIDS in their families will face custody changes. It is crucial that these children move into their second families in a minimally traumatic way. To ensure this, the law must: (a) implement fully a broadened definition of *family;* (b) help the child maintain continuity in relationships; and (c) provide better support to the child's new family. Excellent analyses exist of the difficult legal and emotional issues concerning custody and placement.[4] This section highlights, from a slightly broader legal perspective, several issues of particular importance to children living in families with AIDS.

Implementing a Broadened Definition of "Family"

The Constitution of the United States protects the "sanctity" of the family and shields from unnecessary governmental interference the essential role of parents in the custody, care and nurture of their children. What constitutes a family entitled to constitutional protection is not limited by the United States Supreme Court to the traditional "nuclear" family, and the definition of family has expanded over time. In *Moore v. City of East Cleveland* the Court held invalid in 1977 a definition of *family* in a zoning ordinance that made it unlawful for a grandmother to live in a single household with her son and her two grandsons, one of whom had been orphaned by the death of his mother.[5] The Court explained: "Ours is by no means a tradition limited to respect for the bonds uniting the members of the nuclear family. The tradition of uncles, aunts, cousins, and especially grandparents sharing a household along with parents and children has roots equally venerable and equally deserving of constitutional recognition. Over the years millions of our citizens have grown up in just such an environment, and most, surely, have profited from it. . . . Especially in times of adversity, such as the death of a spouse or economic need, the broader family has tended to come together for mutual sustenance and to maintain or rebuild a secure home life."[6]

Though courts often stress that biological relationships are central to the definition of family, the Supreme Court has stated clearly that "biological relationships are not exclusive determinants of the existence of a family."[7] A family is also created by law (through marriage and adoption) and is, increasingly, defined by function. As the Court explained in *Smith v. OFFER,* "The importance of the familial relationship, to the individual involved and to the society, stems from the emotional attachments that derive from the intimacy of daily association, and from the role it plays in 'promot[ing] a way of life' through the instruction of children."[8] Courts have come to view responsibility, dependency, and relationships of deep emotional significance as key to this functional definition.

Some federal statutes that promise supportive services to families also explicitly embrace a broadened definition of the term. The 1993 Omnibus Budget Reconciliation Act (OBRA), for example, created a new but fiscally capped program, the Family Preservation and Support Services Program (subpart 2 of Title IV-B of the Social Security Act).[9] Its preventive, community-based family support and family preservation services explicitly are established to benefit children living in "extended" as well as foster and adoptive families.[10] OBRA was passed to help states fulfill the "reasonable efforts" requirement of the federal Adoption Assistance and Child Welfare Act of 1980 (AACWA).[11] AACWA, by its text and legislative history, requires each state (as a prerequisite to receiving federal reimbursement for foster care expenses) to make "reasonable efforts" to maintain the child with his or her family—specifying parents so long as they are able to meet the child's needs, but including other "family" when the parents can no longer care for him or her. No precise definition of *reasonable efforts* exists, but the requirement has been interpreted to include such things as: (*a*) a thorough assessment of the family's needs and eligibility for various benefit programs; (*b*) high-quality, well-coordinated services that are targeted to meet family need and are easily accessible to the family (counseling for all family members, homemaking services, temporary child care, transportation assistance, intensive family preservation services); and (*c*) well-trained child welfare workers to assist the family.[12]

Though the AACWA's "reasonable efforts" requirement embraces a broad definition of family, insufficient funding for family support and preservation services often results in a child's placement out of his family.[13] OBRA's $1 billion in new funds over five years cannot meet projected demand and the financially capped program perpetuates the system of financial incentives that favors foster care expenditures (which have open-ended funding) over expenditures to avert foster placements. Unfortunately, the United States Supreme Court decided in *Suter v. Artist M.* that the "reasonable efforts" requirement neither confers an enforceable private right on its beneficiaries nor creates an implied cause of action on their behalf.[14] Thus, until a private right of action is restored by Congress, parents and children who would benefit from full enforcement of this requirement are prevented from bringing suit to compel states to comply with it.

Necessary Changes

The emergence of AIDS poses a challenge to the law: to implement its expanding definition of *family* in a manner that serves the interests of children who are losing parents and family members to the disease.

• The law's definition of *family* must recognize and accommodate ethnic and cultural differences (as required by the constitutional guarantee of equal protection and by statutes prohibiting discrimination on the basis of race, ethnicity, and national origin). For children being orphaned by AIDS, family should be defined from the child's point of view, including those persons, unrelated as well as related, with whom a child lives and on whom he or she relies to satisfy physical and emotional needs as the parents' ability to do so wanes.

• The "reasonable efforts" requirement of the AACWA must be fully implemented. Sufficient government funds must be allocated to provide family support and preservation services to extended, foster, and adoptive families as well as birth families. A private right of action to enforce compliance with this requirement must be restored.

Maintaining Continuity in the Child's Relationships

Relationships with the Ill Parents

Challenges to a child's right to continue to reside with a parent infected with HIV arise generally in two contexts: (*a*) custody disputes between family members and (*b*) state dependency proceedings. In the former, a healthy noncustodial parent (or other relative) may claim it is not in the best interests of a child to remain in the custody of (or even visit with) an infected parent. In the latter, the state may seek to remove a child from the home to protect him or her from harm.

In both contexts, fear of casual transmission of the virus from parent to child is rejected uniformly as a basis for changing custody. Similarly, without an individualized determination of incapacity to meet the child's needs, the mere fact that a parent has HIV infection is no grounds for change. Attempts to shield a child from the emotional pain of watching an ill parent slowly die also have been rejected as a reason to restrict contact.[15]

When parents become so ill they can no longer provide care to their children, the state may become involved. The constitutional protection afforded families restricts the state's power to remove children from their parents to instances of demonstrated abuse, neglect, or abandonment. As noted above, the state has certain affirmative statutory obligations under AACWA, still not fully honored, to offer and provide assistance to keep children within their families rather than removing them into foster care placements with strangers.

Facilitating Planned Transitions to New Caregivers

Because the course of HIV disease is distinguished by episodes of acute, incapacitating illness that are unpredictable in their onset and resolution, temporary transitions to substitute caregivers may be necessary while the parents are living with the disease. Also, many children living with parents who have HIV disease will need to make a transition to a second family when their parents die. At these points, it is important that disruption and uncertainty be minimized.

Unfortunately, the fit between current laws governing custody and guardianship and the needs of families living with HIV disease is a poor one. Current law fails to provide appropriate mechanisms for shifting responsibility for care of children during periods of temporary parental incapacity. The law assumes that when one parent is ill or dies, the other parent is able and willing to provide care, a false assumption if the other parent is absent or has already become ill or died from AIDS. The law works slowly, leaving children with a sense of prolonged uncertainty about their future placement. Finally, the law generally assumes some nongovernmental means of family support. In families for whom government benefits are a primary means of financial support, changes in custody of a child can trigger a decrease in parents' income and benefits, which can undermine the well-being of all involved.

A parent living with HIV disease who cannot rely on the other parent for future care of their child has a number of imperfect options under current law in most states. Each has some advantages; all have problems.

Informal arrangements. A simple option is the informal arrangement, which is easily accomplished but fails to transfer sufficient legal authority to a new caregiver and can limit sources of governmental support for the child.

A power of attorney. Execution of a power of attorney is sometimes useful to transfer legal authority and even grant an unrelated person temporary custody without going to court, but it may not be recognized as legally valid. It also may be time-limited and require periodic renewal, limiting its usefulness when a parent has episodic lapses in capacity.

Designation of a guardian in a will. A will is a quick and relatively easy way to designate a guardian for one's children after one's death. Wills are far superior to having no custody plan but are risky because: (*a*) the transfer of guardianship occurs after death; (*b*) delays in probating the will may result in a child's temporary placement in foster care; (*c*) there is no guarantee that the court will approve the parent's choice of guardian when deciding what serves the "best interests" of the child, and if the court questions the choice, the parent will be unavailable to explain it; and (*d*) in some states, the designation of a guardian in a will is invalid if the child's other parent is still alive (even if the surviving parent cannot be located, has had no contact with the child, or would be an unfit caretaker).

Appointment of a guardian before death. Though most states require that a parent have died before a new guardian is appointed, a few allow appointment of a guardian before death. This option can be emotionally wrenching because a parent typically must relinquish parental rights and responsibilities once the guardian is appointed by the court, even though the parent is still willing and able to provide care. It is also a risky strategy because guardian status lacks legal permanence and the court is not required to appoint the parent's or child's choice of guardian.

Arranged adoption. The safest option in terms of assuring a permanent placement is arranged adoption, but it is emotionally difficult for the same reasons as the appointment of a guardian before death: the adoption order terminates the parents' legal rights and responsibilities. It also requires court approval of the adoptive parents. Some parents may choose to initiate proceedings while they are alive but to defer final action until after their deaths. Others who try to complete the adoption before their deaths may seek rights to some continuing contact with the child, sometimes through an informal agreement with the adopting parents (an "open" adoption).

Voluntary placement into foster care. The best option may be foster care if family members are willing to care for the children but need assistance to do so. In states with "kinship foster care" (for example, New York, Illinois, California), a parent can request placement with relatives, and the relatives, when approved, then receive monthly foster care payments for care of children eligible for federally funded foster care, as well as supportive social services.[16] This option also has risks: (*a*) voluntary placement represents surrender of legal custody to the state; (*b*) the state must approve the relative home and may place the child with strangers until approval is completed; and (*c*) voluntary placements in foster care can be time-limited.[17] In addition, the state will continue to monitor the relative's home, an intrusion that many resent, though one that may serve the best interests of the child in some circumstances.

Involuntary placement into foster care. If the parent becomes incapable of meeting the child's needs before making a formal custody plan, involuntary foster care placement is a likely result. For many children from families affected by AIDS, foster care poses potential risks, including:

- Difficulty finding foster placements able and willing to accept sibling groups, resulting in further fracture of family bonds.
- Placements distant from siblings, other family and friends, and community.
- A lengthy future in foster care, because most states now fail to move children quickly from foster homes into permanent placements with adoptive parents, especially older children for whom adoptive placements may be hard

to find or inappropriate. The child often drifts from one temporary placement to another until he or she "ages out," with little support for independent living.

Systemic problems—inadequate funding, caseloads increasing in size and complexity, an insufficient number of placement alternatives appropriate to children's needs—plague virtually all foster care systems in the country. Foster care drift is a particular danger for children who resemble those most likely to be orphaned by AIDS (older children, for example, those with more than two siblings, those with emotional or adjustment problems). Its danger is exacerbated by the children's status as orphans. With no parent available to challenge state decisions, these children risk becoming orphans within our legal system as well. All children who are the subject of dependency proceedings need independent representation from the moment the state intervenes in the life of their family until the case is closed (by return to family or adoption). An aggressive advocate, monitoring all state decisions and actions and intervening when necessary, is essential to minimize further harm to children who fall into foster care. Unfortunately, appointment of counsel for these children is discretionary in some states. In other states, counsel is appointed for the dependency proceedings, but the appointment does not continue throughout the eighteen months between federally required judicial reviews of the child's status. Payment for counsel is often so low that the quality of representation can suffer.

Thus, of the seven options discussed, none meets completely the placement planning needs of parents with HIV disease. In particular, all options lack the flexibility necessary for this disease, which, up until the moment of death, causes parental incapacity episodically and unpredictably. To be sure, some formal planning for legal transfer of guardianship (by will, by guardianship petition, through adoption) is far preferable to no planning at all, but families should not have to choose among poor alternatives.

A number of states (among them New York, Florida, Illinois, and Connecticut) have responded to the placement needs of parents living with HIV disease by adopting standby guardian laws. Though these statutes differ in the manner and timing of the standby guardian's appointment, characteristically they explicitly permit the guardianship question to be decided before the parent dies. A parent, while still alive and competent, designates a standby guardian whose authority takes effect at some defined point in the future—when the parent is mentally incapacitated, physically debilitated, consents to transfer of guardianship, or dies. Unlike traditional guardian appointments, these laws do not require the parent to relinquish any parental rights until the moment the parent becomes unable to provide care. Like traditional guardian appointments (and unlike wills), however, the laws allow the court to inquire into the background of the proposed guardian and the child's best interests before the parent's incapacity or death and thereby have the benefit of the parent's insights about the best care plan for the child. As currently written, such laws do not consistently ensure that the appointment preserves eligibility for benefits that might otherwise be available to the child and the new guardian, and the laws often require court involvement even if there is no dispute.

Maintaining the New Families

To reduce the possibility of further disruption in the lives of children orphaned by AIDS, it is essential that their new families be supported. Federal law provides adoption subsidies for children with "special needs" who are eligible for federally funded foster care. "Special needs" include factors that might make it difficult for a child to be adopted without financial assistance, like ethnic background, age, membership in a sibling group, or medical conditions or disabilities.[18] The subsidy includes the parents' nonrecurring adoption expenses, a monthly allowance for support (for which there is no means test imposed on the adoptive parents), and Medicaid eligibility for the child (whether or not the child actually receives an adoption subsidy payment). Unfortunately, in many states the foster care payment exceeds the adoption subsidy, creating financial disincentives to adopt.[19] In addition, postadoptive services can be essential, and are required (though not uniformly provided) in all states under AACWA. They can include respite care, support groups for parents and children, intensive family preservation services, and parenting skills classes emphasizing behavior management for problems experienced by many children who are adopted when older.

Necessary Changes

The following three changes can improve markedly the law's responsiveness to children affected by AIDS who are facing changes in guardianship and custody:

- Adopting "standby" guardian laws that allow authority to vest in a standby guardian at times of parental incapacity, assure that the authority returns to the parent in times of wellness, preserve entitlements to benefits, allow appointment of a standby guardian after the filing parent has made reasonable attempts to provide notice to an absent parent (though without prejudice to the rights of the absent parent), and require court involvement only in the event of a dispute.
- Mandating that each state provide representation for a child from the beginning to the end of state involvement with that child and his family, at a rate of compensation sufficient to attract competent, trained counsel, and expediting all judicial proceedings.

• Mandating that adoption assistance subsidies equal the rate paid for foster care, so foster parents (relative or otherwise) are not penalized financially for adopting a child.

Ensuring the Health of the Surviving Children

Children and youths who survive AIDS in their families face substantial threats to their own health. Many require well-child care, their health needs having been subordinated to the health needs of ill family members. Many require mental health services as they learn to cope with their extraordinary losses. Youths orphaned by AIDS who strike out on their own, without means of support, may engage in survival sex—the exchange of sex for money, food, drugs, or a place to sleep—exposing them to risk of HIV and other sexually transmitted diseases. Others may turn to drugs and alcohol. As earlier chapters note, teen pregnancies, declining school performance, and acting out behaviors are common among these adolescents. This conduct mirrors a variety of other behaviors that may pose high risk of transmission of HIV, a risk that increases as the prevalence of HIV infections among United States youths increases.

To ensure the health of these surviving children, the law must reduce those barriers to care over which it has some influence. This section discusses two such barriers: (*a*) restrictions on a minor's right to consent to health care, and (*b*) the actual availability of health care for children and youth.

Eliminating Restrictions on a Minor's Right to Consent to Health Care

Though all adolescents are adversely affected by restrictions on a minor's right to consent to health care, this barrier may be especially great for AIDS-affected youths. These youths may be reluctant to seek parental consent lest they burden their ill parents with knowledge of *their* health problems. They may not feel comfortable confiding in a new guardian, especially about sensitive matters. The state may be their lawful guardian, or they may have run away from home and have no available legal guardian. The law's lack of clarity about their rights must be corrected.

Minors generally lack legal capacity to consent; permission of a parent or guardian is required. However, courts and legislatures have created an increasing number of exceptions that grant minors a limited right to consent. These exceptions vary by state and may be based on a variety of factors, including the minor's financial, housing, and marital status ("emancipated" and married minors can consent); the minor's maturity; or a need for emergency care. In addition, state and federal statutes allow minors of varying ages to consent to treatment for certain socially sensitive medical conditions (for example, diagnosis and treatment of STDs and other communicable diseases, family planning services, and, increasingly, substance abuse treatment, mental health care, and testing for HIV).[20] Minors also have a constitutional right to privacy in making decisions about reproductive health care, including decisions about contraception and abortion.[21] Although a minor's right to receive abortion services without parental approval is often more limited than the right to receive contraceptives, courts require that abortion statutes restricting a minor's right to consent give her the option of avoiding parental involvement through a confidential and expeditious judicial bypass procedure.[22]

Much uncertainty about minors' rights persists. The law concerning HIV testing and treatment is illustrative. An increasing number of states (at least twenty) have statutes that explicitly allow minors to consent to their own HIV tests. Some cover minors of any age, while others set a minimum age, often twelve years old.[23] Some link capacity to consent to the minor's ability to understand the care to be provided, regardless of age. Some require both a minimum age and evidence of maturity to make an informed decision. Some implicitly authorize consent by permitting minors to consent to diagnosis and treatment for a communicable and/or sexually transmitted disease and classifying HIV as such. Many of the statutes that explicitly or implicitly grant minors permission to consent to tests for HIV, however, are silent about a number of important and related issues, including: (a) the minor's capacity to give consent for any needed treatment; (b) whether the right to consent to care also includes the right to refuse care (a particularly difficult issue if the parents want the minor treated or the child is a ward of the state); and (c) whether the parents can, or must, be notified when the minor seeks and receives care.

Necessary Changes

With ambiguity in the law, liability-conscious health care providers will likely err on the side of refusing to care for minors without parental consent.[24] Clarity is essential, as is recognition that those adolescents who feel comfortable involving adults generally will do so, while those who do not should nonetheless be able to receive care. Each state should enact legislation that:

- Grants minors who are mature enough to seek health care on their own the legal capacity to grant consent to that care and to withhold consent to unwanted care. Such statutes must explicitly include not only minors who are living with parents or legal guardians but also those who are in state custody.
- Protects the confidentiality of this encounter between the minor and the health care system.

Several "model" minor's consent statutes exist, including the Pediatric Bill of Rights (drafted by the National Center for the Prevention and Treatment of Child Abuse and Neglect and adopted by the Board of Trustees of the National Association of Children's Hospitals and Related Institutions) and the Model Act Providing for Consent of Minors for Health Services (approved by the Council on Child Health of the American Academy of Pediatrics).[25] They can provide a useful starting point for reform. By clarifying the law of consent for all adolescents, this formidable barrier to health care for HIV-affected youths will be addressed as well.

Increasing Access to Health Care

Our current health care system fails many of our children and youths. As of 1993, 12.4 percent of children under eighteen had no health insurance, public or private: 12.0 percent of all white children; 13.5 percent of African-American children, and 25.7 percent of Latino children.[26] In such cases, family resources often go first to the care of ill family members rather than well children. Barriers to care can exist even for those minors living in insured families if the minor seeks care without the consent or knowledge of a parent or guardian. Children in state custody, entitled to health care at state expense, too often also fail to receive appropriate care.

Increasing health care access for all children and youths will necessarily benefit those children from families living with HIV disease. Conversely, the significant health needs of children affected by HIV provide a discrete target for improvements in our system from which other children may also benefit. This section briefly highlights four ways in which the delivery of health care to these children may be enhanced.

Medicaid. Given the current demographics of the epidemic, many children from families living with HIV disease are eligible for Medicaid and therefore entitled to all services required by its Early and Periodic Screening, Diagnosis, and Treatment program (EPSDT), one of the most comprehensive health benefit plans in the country. EPSDT requires, for example, periodic and comprehensive health screenings and assessments (including developmental and mental health status assessments), all health care services (whether optional or mandatory under Medicaid law) that are necessary to diagnose and treat identified health problems, and a broad range of enabling services (outreach, case management, transportation, and scheduling assistance, for example). The promise of EPSDT, however, remains unfulfilled in most states. Low provider fees (resulting in poor provider participation) and state failures to fully implement EPSDT's comprehensive requirements (including its outreach requirements) limit eligible children's access to care. In addition, fewer than 60 percent of children who are eligible for Medicaid on the basis of family income are actually receiving Medicaid services.[27] Child advocates are

increasingly pursuing litigation to compel states to comply with these extensive federal mandates, and this litigation is meeting with significant success.[28]

New private insurance mandates. For orphaned children now living in
families who have private health insurance, the 1993 OBRA mandates significant new access to health coverage. It requires group health plans to cover
children placed for adoption in families with existing private health insurance
(whether or not adoption has become final), just as such plans must now
cover the family's biological children. Plans also cannot deny health care coverage for an adoptive child based on a preexisting condition.

Children and youths in state custody. Children affected by HIV who come
into state custody (through the foster care or juvenile justice systems, for
example) have a constitutional right to medical and mental health care.[29] In
addition, children in foster care have statutory rights to health care under the
federal Adoption Assistance and Child Welfare Act of 1980. Since the early
1980s, child advocates have used litigation to force states to meet this legal
obligation to foster children, with significant success (in Illinois, Connecticut,
Maryland, Missouri, Washington, D.C., and Arkansas, for example).[30] Often,
Child Welfare League Standards for Health Care Services for Children in
Out-of-Home Care are adopted as the required standard for care imposed on
the state.[31] Other court decisions have mandated improvements in health care
for children and youths in juvenile correctional settings.

School-based health care. The United States has a long history of providing some health and social services to children in the public school setting.[32] Community-based institutions whose skilled staff have frequent
contact with virtually all children and their families, schools are prime sites
for providing confidential, easily accessible, comprehensive health education
and medical and mental health services to children and youths. Unfortunately, too few schools accept the challenge.[33] Two issues within the debate
concerning the role of schools in providing a full continuum of health care are
pertinent to this discussion: (*a*) what sort of health education should be provided to students and (*b*) whether the provision of primary care services
within a school setting is consistent with its educational role—and, if it is,
what types of services should be provided. A vocal minority of parents advocates censorship as a response to these issues. Often school boards and legislatures respond by restricting the content of health education and services.

Though state directives to provide sexuality and AIDS education in the
schools are common, censorship efforts often compromise the comprehen-
siveness and accuracy of the education provided.[34] In one 1993 survey, 92 percent of the states reported controversies at the local level regarding

implementation of sexuality education.[35] In some instances, discussion of certain topics, like abortion, is banned. In others, particular viewpoints are banned or a particular viewpoint must be emphasized. Often instruction is not developmentally appropriate and fails to cover the three learning domains (cognitive, affective, and skills).[36] In addition, not all students may actually receive this education; all states with policy about sexuality education and AIDS education give parents the option of excluding their children from some or all of the program. Washington State wisely conditions this "opt-out" on a parent's first attending a meeting to review the curriculum and materials.

Similarly, the idea of distributing condoms in schools evokes a strong censorship response.[37] Some states explicitly forbid distribution of contraceptives on school property. An increasing number of school districts (New York, Philadelphia, the District of Columbia, New Haven, and Los Angeles, for example) include condom distribution as a school health service to help minors gain access to a tool that can decrease risk of HIV, other STDs, and pregnancy. Some of them (New York City and Philadelphia, for example) have had to defend their action against litigation brought by irate parents claiming infringement of their constitutional rights to exercise their religion and to direct the upbringing of their children. Not all minors have access to this service even in those districts that have established it; some programs require parental permission for students to participate, though most require that objecting parents request exclusion.

Efforts to censor the content of health education and services in our schools (by suit or mere threat of suit) are problematic in at least three respects.

First, such censorship is not favored by the majority of the public. National polls demonstrate substantial support for explicit school-based AIDS education and prevention programs. Ninety-three percent of persons polled in a 1991 Roper poll favored AIDS education for elementary school students, and 81 percent thought that "pretty explicit sexual material" is needed to teach teenagers adequately about HIV. National polls also indicate increasing support for condom distribution in high schools (with the proportion who favor distribution increasing from 37 percent in 1988 to at least 63 percent in 1991 and 1992).[38]

Second, censorship efforts thwart effective health interventions. Notwithstanding their current shortcomings, school-based AIDS education programs appear already to be reducing some of the adolescent behaviors that pose risk of HIV transmission. The 1994 report of the Centers for Disease Control and Prevention's 1989 and 1990 national surveys of students in grades 9–12 found a significant increase in school-based HIV instruction, an associated increase in HIV knowledge, and a statistically significant decrease among some subgroups of students in certain HIV-related behaviors (having multiple sexual partners, injecting illicit drugs).[39]

Third, censorship efforts may be unlawful. Courts repeatedly invalidate efforts by school officials and by parents to promote one viewpoint and exclude others on controversial matters in school curricula and in the selection of books for school libraries. They reject the imposition of a "pall of orthodoxy" and the purposeful suppression of ideas, as well as requirements to teach information that is misleading or factually incorrect. For example, a New York City school board resolution that required all AIDS prevention education to devote "substantially" more time and attention to abstinence than to other methods of prevention was ruled unlawful because it violated state regulations protecting academic freedom and threatened the public health by preventing students from receiving accurate and effective health education.[40]

On the other hand, courts remain sympathetic to parents' claims that they have a constitutional right to exclude their children from being exposed in school to certain types of material they find offensive. An intermediate appellate court in New York, for example, found parental involvement provisions to be a prerequisite to a constitutionally valid condom distribution program.[41] Such continued deference to parental authority must be questioned in light of recent expansions in minors' rights to consent to health care for the consequences of unprotected sexual intercourse—and in light of the life-threatening health risks that youth now face.

Just as the law has denied parents, on constitutional grounds, an absolute veto power over their children's decisions about abortion, so too must the law be changed to deny parents an absolute veto over their children's constitutional rights to receive health and life-saving information. Neither should the law afford a vocal minority of parents a veto over the health education and health care provided to children other than their own, allowing their strident objections to reduce prevention messages to a "least offensive" common denominator. AIDS threatens a generation of youths. Without an effective vaccine for HIV disease, education is our only—admittedly imperfect—"vaccine." Effectiveness, not offensiveness, must be the standard by which courts judge such programs.

Necessary Changes

To protect the health of children and youths surviving AIDS in their families (assuming no fundamental change in our health care system that ensures universal access for all children to EPSDT-equivalent health services), the following steps are essential:

- Further expansion of children's eligibility for Medicaid (because EPSDT requires such comprehensive services) and rigorous enforcement of Medicaid mandates.
- Implementation of comprehensive, skills-based, accurate, effective, and developmentally and culturally appropriate health education programs in schools, and in all other sites that provide care to youths: juvenile justice facilities, residential facilities, shelters, group homes, and government-funded community agencies. To encourage states to amend their laws to require such programs, the federal government should condition states' receipt of federal health education funds on existence of such requirements or provide financial incentives for such changes.
- Expansion of school-based health clinics to reduce barriers to care for students who are uninsured, or who wish confidential health services.
- Adoption of state statutes and policy that allow adolescents to receive, on their own consent, school-based health education and health services and that require parents to view the health education curriculum before they can withdraw a younger child from the program.
- Adoption of state statutes that clarify that schools not only have authority to provide condom distribution programs but also should do so.
- Implementation of public health education efforts that are targeted at out-of-school youths and are free of unconstitutionally vague content censorship by the government sponsor.

In *The Plague*, Albert Camus writes, "All I maintain is that on this earth there are pestilences and there are victims, and it's up to us, so far as possible, not to join forces with the pestilences. That may sound simple to the point of childishness; I can't judge if it's simple, but I know it's true. . . . I grant we should add a third category: that of the true healers. But it's a fact one doesn't come across many of them, and anyhow it must be a hard vocation. That's why I decided to take, in every predicament, the victims' side, so as to reduce the damage done. Among them I can at least try to discover how one attains to the third category; in other words, to peace."[42] In the AIDS pandemic, the law cannot be a true healer, and it risks joining forces with the pestilences—when it presents families confronting HIV disease with no good choices for custody planning, when it perpetuates a health care system that delays and denies essential care to those in need, when it closes its eyes to discrimination. A clear alternative exists. The law, and all those working within it, must reduce the damage done. All must take the side of families struggling with HIV disease and the forgotten children within them whose childhoods will forever be transformed by the many deaths in their families.

Notes

1. Bowleg, L., and K. Cauley, 1992, *A policymaker's guide on HIV/AIDS for the 1990s*, Washington, D.C.: Intergovernmental Health Policy Project, George Washington University; Bowleg, L., 1993, *A summary of HIV/AIDS laws from the 1992 state legislative sessions*, Wash-

ington, D.C.: Intergovernmental Health Policy Project, George Washington University; Bowleg, L., 1994, *A summary of HIV/AIDS laws from the 1993 legislative session,* Washington, D.C.: Intergovernmental Health Policy Project.

2. Bowleg and Cauley, see note 1 above.

3. Illinois, for example, requires that whenever a school-aged child is reported to the health department as having HIV disease, the department must give "prompt and confidential notice" to the principal of the child's school and to the school superintendent. The principal "may, as necessary" disclose the child's identity to the school nurse, her classroom teachers, and persons required by state and federal law to decide her placement or educational program. The principal also may inform "such other persons as may be necessary that an infected child is enrolled at that school, so long as the child's identity is not revealed." 410 Illinois Consolidated Statutes § 315/2a (1993). Missouri conditions such mandatory disclosure on the school's first adopting a policy consistent with CDC recommendations "on school children who test positive for HIV." Revised Statutes of Missouri, § 191.689 (1993).

4. Soler, M., et al., 1989, *Representing the child client,* New York: Matthew Bender; Schulman, I., and R. Behrman, eds., 1993, *Adoption: The Future of Children* 3 (1), Los Altos, Calif.: The David and Lucille Packard Foundation; Cooper, E., 1992, HIV-infected parents and the law: Issues of custody, visitation, and guardianship. In *AIDS agenda: Emerging issues in civil rights,* ed. N. D. Hunter and W. B. Rubenstein, New York: New Press, 69–117; English, A., 1992, The HIV-AIDS epidemic and the child welfare system: Protecting the rights of infants, young children, and adolescents, *Iowa Law Review* 77 (4): 1509–1560; Banks, T. L., 1993, Reproduction and parenting, in *AIDS law today: A new guide to the public,* ed. S. Burris, H. L. Dalton, and J. L. Miller, New Haven: Yale University Press, 216–241; Pinott, M., 1993, Custody and placement: The legal issues. In *Orphans of the HIV epidemic,* ed. C. Levine, New York: United Hospital Fund, 75–84; Legal Analysis, 1993, Standby guardianship: A promising option for ailing parents? *American Bar Association Juvenile and Child Welfare Law Reporter* 12: 110–112.

5. *Moore v. City of East Cleveland,* 421 U.S. 494, 504 (1977).

6. *Moore v. City of East Cleveland,* 421 U.S. 504–505.

7. *Smith v. OFFER* 431 U.S. 816, 843 (1977).

8. *Smith v. OFFER,* 431 U.S. 843.

9. Public Law 103-66.

10. Family support services are defined as "community-based services to promote well-being of children and families designed to increase the strength and stability of families (including adoptive, foster, and extended families), . . . to afford children a stable and supportive family environment, and to otherwise enhance child development." They can include home visits, parent support groups, respite care, structured activities to improve parent-child relationships, drop-in family centers, information and referral services, and early developmental screening of children to assess their need for specific services.

Family preservation services are defined broadly as "services for children and families designed to help families (including adoptive and extended families) at risk or in crisis." They can include programs to promote a planned permanent living arrangement; preplacement preventive services programs (such as counseling; financial assistance for food, utility bills, and housing; help obtaining public benefits; child care assistance; homemaker services; and intensive family preservation programs); aftercare services for children returned to their families from foster care; and respite care for caregivers. Because of limited funding, many states restrict eligibility to children who are at "imminent risk of placement" in foster care and whose families are willing to try a family preservation program as an alternative to such placement.

11. The AACWA requires each state that seeks federal reimbursement for a portion of its foster

care and adoption assistance payments to prepare a state plan that meets federal requirements. One of these requirements is that the state will make "reasonable efforts" before placing a child in foster care to prevent or eliminate the need for removal of the child from his home, and again after a placement to return the child home. 42 U.S.C. § 671 (a)(15).

12. Goodman, S., and J. Hurley, 1993, *Reasonable efforts: Who decides what's reasonable?* (a paper commissioned by the United States Department of Health and Human Services, Office of the Assistant Secretary for Planning and Evaluation). Some courts have required child welfare agencies to provide assistance to families in obtaining adequate housing. See, for example, *In the matter of Enrique R.,* 494 N.Y.S. 2d 800 (N.Y. Fam. Ct. 1985) (where the child was not released from foster care to live with grandmother solely because she lacked adequate housing, agency must assist grandmother in obtaining housing, including taking legal action on the grandmother's behalf to secure a preference in tenant selection for public housing). See A. Shotton, 1990, State appellate courts move toward definition of "reasonable efforts," *Youth Law News* 11 (3): 1–6.

13. Inadequate funding for family preservation services has caused some states to rely on creative funding strategies to augment the programs (for example, classifying family preservation services as "health related assessment and treatment" services that can receive federal reimbursement under Medicaid/EPSDT, or adopting a voluntary cap on federal Title IV-E foster care funds and then transferring money that is not spent on foster care payments to the state's Title IV-B account for family preservation services).

14. *Suter v. Artist M.,* 112 S. Ct. 1360 (1992).

15. A New York court, for example, refused to terminate the custodial rights of an infected parent on this basis, stating that "even if the respondent . . . had a shortened life span, this fact would not justify removing children from their long-term custodial parent with whom they have such strong bonds of love and affection." *Doe v. Roe,* 526 N.Y.S. 2d 718 (N.Y. Sup. Ct. 1988).

16. *Kinship foster care,* as used here, refers to formal kinship foster care in which a child, in the legal custody of the state child welfare agency, lives in a relative's home that has been licensed or otherwise approved by the agency. These kin provide the child with full-time care, must work with the state on a permanency plan for the child, and receive financial assistance through foster care payments. Informal kinship care arrangements also exist in many families but do not afford kin caregivers an equivalent right to foster care payments, which typically far exceed AFDC benefits. Kinship foster care differs from standby guardianship (discussed later) though both may be useful for HIV-infected parents during acute episodes of illness and hospitalizations; both provide a way for others to assume temporary custody of their children. In kinship foster care, the state itself assumes legal custody of the children during these times of parental incapacity, and the state can request a court to continue this custody if it has evidence that the child is uncared for, even after the parent regains health and seeks an end to the voluntary placement.

States are constitutionally required to allow "kin" to be foster parents, though not all do so. The United States Supreme Court held in *Miller v. Youakim,* 440 U.S. 125 (1979), that it is unconstitutional for states to deny foster care benefits to children who meet the requirements of Title IV-E of the Social Security Act solely because they are placed in the home of a relative. In *Lipscomb v. Simmons,* 884 F. 2d. 1242 (9th Cir. 1989), two of three children in a family were placed in foster care with strangers because a relative was financially unable to meet the needs of all three siblings. The court decided that the children had a constitutionally protected liberty interest in living with family members and that the state had an obligation to protect that interest by providing foster care benefits to the relative. Children in kin foster placements are also entitled to supportive foster care services. For example, the 1988 consent decree in *L.J. v. Massinga,* 699 F. Supp. 508 (D. Md. 1988), was modified in 1991 to ensure that most of the original consent judgment provisions, which expanded treatment and services, would be extended to foster children placed with relatives in unlicensed care, 778 F. Supp. 253 (1991). Unfortunately, to avoid providing supportive services and paying foster care rates, some states fail to inform relatives of their right to become foster parents and/or try to coerce them into becoming private guardians (by telling the relatives, for example, that unless they accept appointment as private guardians the child will be placed in a nonrelative home). At least one recent case challenged these practices explicitly and forced their change: *Reid v. Suter*, No. 89 J 6195 & 6196 (Cir. Ct., Cook Cty. Ill.) (1992 consent decree requiring agency to: (*a*) identify and assess potential relative placements whenever a child cannot remain with parents; (*b*) give all potential and actual relative caretakers information in a standardized format that describes the legal and financial differences between being a private guardian and being a foster parent before being forced to make a choice between the two; and (*c*) inform relatives about all placement decisions and tell them about the appeal process from those decisions).

17. Some states may waive or alter some of the licensing requirements that are generally applied to foster parents; physical size and space requirements may be less stringent, for example, and there may be expedited emergency approval processes for relative placements.

18. Each state defines what constitutes "special needs" based on that state's experience with barriers to adoptive placements without assistance. Some states explicitly define the term in statute or policy; others leave great discretion to the child welfare agency. Useful discussions of special needs adoption assistance are found in A. Bussiere, 1993, Adoption assistance taking on greater importance in quest for permanence, *Youth Law News* 14 (6): 1–6; McKenzie, J., 1993, Adoption of children with special needs; and in Schulman and Behrman, see note 4 above.

19. States differ in whether adoption assistance benefits are counted as income in calculating eligibility for other programs (for example, SSI, AFDC, medical assistance, food stamps, public housing). As a result, adopting families in some states may have their benefits decreased or may become ineligible for a program if they accept an adoption subsidy — yet another disincentive to adoption.

20. For example, sections of the Social Security Act governing AFDC and Medicaid require that confidential family planning services be provided to all eligible recipients, including sexually active minors [42 U.S.C. § 602 (a)(15), § 1396d (a)(4)(C)]. Title X of the Public Health Service Act, the largest source of federal funding for family planning programs in the United States, mandates that teenagers receive confidential services [42 U.S.C. § 300 (a); 42 CFR §§ 59.5 (a)(4), 59.15]. Federal courts, which interpret these statutes as requiring that minors be allowed to consent to family planning services, have invalidated both state laws and federal and state regulations that have tried to impose parental/guardian consent or notification requirements on the receipt of such services. See, for example, *Planned Parenthood of Utah v. Dandoy*, 810 F. 2d 984 (10th Cir. 1987) (invalidating Utah law requiring that providers get written parental consent in order to obtain Medicaid reimbursement for contraceptive services given to unemancipated minors); *Planned Parenthood Federation of America v. Heckler*, 712 F. 2d 650 (D.C. Cir. 1983) (invalidating, under Title X, federal regulations which required that parents be notified of family planning services provided to otherwise eligible minors); *Doe v. Irwin*, 615 F. 2d 1162 (6th Cir. 1980), *cert. denied*, 449 U.S. 829 (1980) (rejecting parents' claim that they had a constitutional right to be notified before prescription contraceptives were distributed to their minor daughters). Nearly every state by statute allows minors to consent to treatment for sexually transmitted diseases. Horowitz, R., and H. Davidson, 1984, *Legal rights of children*, § 4.14, Colorado Springs: Shepard's/McGraw-Hill. Many states extend minors' consent authority to other conditions listed in the text. See A. Elster and N. Kuznets, 1994, *AMA guidelines for adolescent preventive services (GAPS): Recommendations and rationale*, Baltimore: Williams and Wilkins, which discusses current state law, the importance of ensuring confidential health services for adolescents, and the "strong national consensus" supporting this position, p. 7. Some states limit the mental health treatment that can be provided to a minor before parental consent or notification is required. See,

for example, Connecticut General Statutes § 19a-14c (1992); Ohio Revised Code § 5122.04 (1994) (six sessions or thirty days).

21. Minors' constitutional right to privacy includes the right to possess and use contraceptives. *Carey v. Population Services, Int.,* 431 U.S. 678 (1977); *Planned Parenthood Association of Utah v. Matheson,* 582 F. Supp. 1001 (D. Utah, 1983) (invalidating a Utah law that required drug stores, physicians, and family planning clinics to notify both parents before giving contraceptives to a minor). Similarly, a minor's decision whether to bear a child or have an abortion is protected by the Constitution against unjustified state intrusion. *Hodgson v. Minnesota,* 497 U.S. 417, 432 (1990).

22. For example, *Belotti v. Baird,* 443 U.S. 622 (1979) (if state requires pregnant minor to obtain one or both parents' consent to an abortion, it must also provide an alternative procedure through which minor can demonstrate that she is mature enough to consent or the abortion is in her best interest); *Hodgson v. Minnesota,* 497 U.S. 417 (1990) (two-parent notification requirement must also have judicial bypass). A number of courts have held that a minor's decision to seek the advice of an attorney and to use the judicial bypass procedure may, in itself, demonstrate sufficient maturity to warrant a finding that the minor is mature enough to consent to an abortion. See, for example, *Ex parte Anonymous,* 595 So. 2d 497 (Ala. 1992).

23. Research shows that adolescents, on average, are indistinguishable from adults in their ability to understand the benefits and risks of treatment options, and to make and express reasonable choices among treatment alternatives. The decision-making process itself has beneficial effects on adolescents, including the enhancement of their compliance with treatment. Melton, G., G. Koocher, and M. Saks, eds., 1993, *Children's competence to consent,* New York: Plenum.

24. No physician has been successfully sued for providing nonnegligent care to a minor without his parent's consent (Elster and Kuznets, see note 20 above, p. 7), so this caution may seem unwarranted. The mere threat of costly litigation, however, often is sufficient to limit minors' access to confidential care.

25. The Pediatric Bill of Rights is reprinted and critiqued in G. E. Raitt, 1975, The minor's right to consent to medical treatment: A corollary of the constitutional right of privacy, *Southern California Law Review* 48: 1417–1456. Committee on Youth, American Academy of Pediatrics, 1973, A model act providing for consent of minors for health services, *Pediatrics* 51: 293–296. Note, however, that this act does not grant minors a right to consent to sterilizations or abortions. The evolution in reproductive rights law in the intervening two decades suggests the importance of a reassessment of its abortion exclusion.

26. United States Census Bureau, 1993, *Current Population Survey* (March). Washington, D.C.: Government Printing Office.

27. National Commission on Children, 1991, *Beyond rhetoric, A new American agenda for children and families,* Washington, D.C.: Government Printing Office, 136. EPSDT requires states to use aggressive outreach to bring more children into care.

28. For example, *Thompson v. Raiford,* No. 3: 92-CV-1939-R (N.D. Texas, Sept. 24, 1993) (order in nationwide class action enforces EPSDT's blood lead testing and monitoring requirement), reprinted in *Medicare and Medicaid Guide (CCH)* ¶ 41,776; *Sanders v. Lewis,* No. 2: 92-0353 (S.D. W. Va., Aug. 16, 1993) (consent decree requires EPSDT outreach and screening of all children in out-of-home placements); *Scott v. Snider,* No. 91-CV-7080 (E.D. Pa. Aug. 11, 1993) (stipulated settlement requires that Medicaid-eligible mothers/infants be informed about EPSDT at time of birth and before discharge from hospital or provider's care); *L.J. v. Massinga,* 699 F. Supp. 508 (D. Md. 1988), *modified,* 778 F. Supp. 253 (1991) (requires timely health screens for foster children).

29. For example, *DeShaney v. Winnebago County Department of Social Services,* 489 U.S. 189, 200 (1989) (state has constitutional obligation to fulfill the basic human needs of any person

in its custody; i.e., it must provide food, clothing, shelter, medical care, and reasonable safety). The government's constitutional duty to provide adequate health care extends to children in foster care. See, for example, *L.J. v. Massinga*, 699 F. Supp. 508 (D. Md. 1988), *aff'd*, 838 F. 2d 188 (4th Cir. 1988), *cert. den.* 488 U.S. 1018 (1989), *modified*, 778 F. Supp. 253 (1991); *G.L. v. Zumwalt*, 564 F. Supp. 1030 (W.D. Mo. 1983) (adequate medical, mental health, and dental care constitutionally required for foster children). The duty to provide health care also extends to children in a correctional setting. Cf., *City of Revere v. Massachusetts General Hospital*, 463 U.S. 239 (1983); *Estelle v. Gamble*, 429 U.S. 97 (1976).

30. For example, *Angela R. v. Clinton*, No. LRC-91-415 (D. Ark. Consent Decree, April 1992); *LaShawn A. v. Dixon*, 762 F. Supp. 959 (D.D.C. 1991); *Juan F. v. O'Neill*, Civ. No. H-89-859 (D. Conn., Consent Decree Jan. 1991); *L.J. v. Massinga*, see note 29 above.

31. E.g., *Angela R. v. Clinton*, see note 30 above; *Juan F. v. O'Neill*, see note 30 above.

32. Tyack, D., 1992, Health and social services in public schools: Historical perspectives. In *School linked services*, ed. R. E. Behrman, Los Altos, Calif.: The David and Lucille Packard Foundation, 19–31.

33. Some schools are implementing school-based grief and loss groups, such as the elementary school grief/loss groups in the San Francisco Public Schools and the elementary school-based bereavement groups organized by the Community Consultation Center at the Henry Street Settlement in New York City. Children may seek or be referred to these groups for help with any type of loss, including HIV-related losses. The Henry Street group found it clinically appropriate to organize three groups: (*1*) for children who had already lost a parent or parents; (*2*) for children anticipating the imminent death of a parent or parents; and (*3*) for children struggling with issues related to living with parents who were chronically or terminally ill. Also, because AIDS-education classes may evoke strong grief reactions among participating children who are living with HIV-related losses in their families, it is essential to link support services for these children to all AIDS educational efforts. How best to treat bereaved children responding to HIV-related losses is a matter for controlled, longitudinal research, as discussed in R. Schilling et al., 1992, Bereavement groups for inner-city children, *Research on Social Work Practice* 2 (3): 405–419, and in G. Zambelli and A. DeRosa, 1992, Bereavement support groups for school-age children: Theory, intervention and case example, *American Journal of Orthopsychiatry* 62 (4): 484–493. Contributors to the June 1994 supplement of *The Journal of Developmental and Behavioral Pediatrics* 15 (3) describe the type of research necessary.

34. According to a 1993 survey of states by the Sex Information and Education Council of the United States (SIECUS), seventeen states mandate sexuality education in their schools, and another thirty encourage it. Local schools, however, have considerable discretion in use of curricula, texts and materials, and only sixteen states monitor the implementation of sexuality education at the local level. Only a minority of states require special certification or training for teachers of sexuality education. SIECUS, 1993, *Unfinished business*, New York: SIECUS. A 1992 SIECUS state survey found that thirty-eight states require AIDS education, and the rest recommend it through statute or policy. Nearly all states provide teacher training and all have advisory groups for program design. SIECUS, 1993, *Future directions: HIV/AIDS education in the nation's schools*, New York: SIECUS.

35. SIECUS, *Unfinished business*, see note 34 above.

36. Ibid.

37. Samuels, S., and M. Smith, 1993, *Condoms in the schools*, Menlo Park, Calif.: The Henry J. Kaiser Family Foundation.

38. Gallup Organization, 1992, Gallup Poll (April 5); Roper Organization, 1991, AIDS: Public attitudes and education needs (June); Kane, Parsons, and Associates, 1988, Parents Magazine-Wave5 poll (January). All three polls are reported in the Poll database in WestLaw.

39. Holtzman, D., et al., 1994, Changes in HIV-related information sources, instruction, knowledge, and behaviors among U.S. high school students, 1989 and 1990, *American Journal of Public Health* 84 (3): 388–393.

40. *Board of Education of New York v. Sobol*, 1993 N.Y. Misc. LEXIS 606 (December 9, 1993).

41. *Alfonso v. Fernandez*, 606 N.Y.S. 2d 259 (1993).

42. Camus, A., 1948, *The plague*, 1991 ed., trans. Stuart Gilbert, New York: Vintage International/Random House.

Chapter 10

Building Child- and Family-Responsive Support Systems

JANICE M. GRUENDEL AND GARY R. ANDERSON

My real name is Joe Louis Lopez. . . . People are afraid of AIDS and you have to show them they're wrong by telling them to read, get their facts right. When I give them the facts about me, people might think, "Oh, get away from him, he has AIDS," but I don't care what they think. It's what I think inside and what my family thinks—my dad, my brothers, and my step-mom, Susan. . . .

I got it because my real mom used to do drugs. She didn't realize it, though. . . . I didn't know my mom was sick until she went into the hospital. She came out in a month but then she got sick again and went to the hospital again. . . . The next morning my grandfather came and said my mother died. Me and my brother Charles started crying when we found out. Charlie was mad, because she died. She was young. . . .

He don't think about it that much, 'cause if he does, his feelings will come back. Charlie is seventeen. He's my real mom's son, before she got AIDS, but not my dad's, and he's not HIV. I have a little baby brother, Matthew, who's almost two. He's Susan and my dad's son, and they're not HIV so he's not either.[1]

Joey, Charlie, and Matthew are real children from a family in which an adult had AIDS. Joey is also infected; Charles and Matthew are affected. We hear the voices of Charlie and Matthew only through the courageous voice of their infected brother, but Charlie and Matthew are not alone in their silence. Before the end of this decade, more than 125,000 children in the United States alone will watch their mothers die of AIDS. Many more—from toddlers to adolescents—will watch other loved ones die as this disease moves from its epicenter in urban areas out into the suburbs and from coastal areas into the heartland of the country.

These will be children born to an infected mother but who escaped infection themselves, or they will be children born before their parent or parents contracted the virus. Some will be their families' only children; others will have several siblings. These siblings may be healthy, or one or more may also be HIV infected. The children may reside in single-parent families, two-parent families, foster and adoptive families, or families reconstituted as the result of divorce or the illness itself. They may live in disadvantaged economic environments or in areas of apparent wealth. They may fail in school and drop out, or they may graduate. They may engage in unsafe behaviors, including unprotected sex and drug use, placing themselves at risk of the very illness that has caused the death of their parents and the fragmentation of their families. Whether from city or suburb, poverty or comfort, whether a toddler or an adolescent, a common bond unites these children: their invisibility in the throes of this unremitting disease within their families, their neighborhoods, and their communities.

Other chapters have presented the developmental, clinical, and legal needs of these children in considerable detail. This chapter explores the major environments from which these children, like all children, receive their social support and suggests ways to modify certain aspects of those systems so they function effectively for children affected by HIV disease. We know already that children affected by HIV will be involved with schools, peers, and other social groups, kinship homes, or alternative living arrangements through the child welfare system. We also know that the social stigma attached to this illness, coupled with the psychological strain resulting from living in families with HIV, can keep affected children from taking advantage of both social and clinical support. Finally, we know that necessary services are not available for many affected children and that even when they are they may not be "child and family friendly."

Before we can begin to identify necessary enhancements within service systems and supportive environments, however, we must reframe the context in which we think about the problems of children and HIV disease. There are six critical issues. First, we must move beyond the medical model as our exclusive reference point for children living in families with HIV. Second, we must work with the broad family system, rather than with the individual alone, as the locus of support efforts. Third, we must understand the needs of HIV-affected children within the context of their general social and cognitive development, from infancy through young adulthood. Fourth, we must apply what is known about resilience—how some children are able to achieve competency while living in extremely disadvantaged circumstances—to our programmatic response to children affected by HIV. Fifth, we must recognize that the needs of these children and their families reflect significant cultural and religious diversity. Finally, we must require that all services be designed to meet the needs of these children and families rather than demanding that children fit into existing categorical structures. Only within this revised frame of reference can we hope to enhance the effectiveness of "helping" systems for children affected by HIV disease and their families.

The first section presents a redefinition of context through brief discussions of each of these six issues. The second section outlines challenges to the formal child welfare, educational, children's mental health, and legal systems. It also describes an expanded role for local community organizations and faith communities, often powerful but overlooked resources for HIV-affected children. The chapter ends by proposing funding and program criteria for policymakers.

Toward a Redefinition of Context

Beyond the Medical Model

Throughout the early course of HIV disease in America, the medical community has been the primary agent of intervention and treatment. In the case of HIV-affected children, however, there are several reasons to involve other systems in the early development of support and intervention. Perhaps most important is the fact that, because these children are not themselves ill, they have remained virtually invisible to the medical system. Second, although children affected by HIV need support and may need clinical intervention, the focus must be on normative development, competence, coping, and resilience. Although the medical system may have the first opportunity to ask about the presence of affected children within families of infected patients, early support for these children will likely need to come from such community-based resources as schools, recreational organizations, and faith communities. When clinical intervention is required, therapeutic services for AIDS-affected children may be most appropriately delivered by community mental health professionals.

This necessary change in perspective—from illness to well-being and from medical to mental health and community support services—actually has its roots within our evolving understanding of HIV disease. Early in the course of this epidemic in America, the medical community and AIDS patients themselves focused on managing the process of "dying of AIDS." More recently, as we have come to understand this disease as a chronic illness progressing over a period of ten to twelve years, the emphasis for infected persons has become "living with AIDS." For children affected by HIV, we must adopt an even more positive objective: "surviving AIDS" and continuing to grow in ways that promote a positive adulthood.

Switching to a reference point that emphasizes wellness and community support for children affected by HIV does not deny the importance of the medical system as the primary provider of services for HIV-infected family members, or as one of the first systems with sufficient information to ask about the presence of affected children in infected families. Nor does it deny the powerful role of a trusted medical adviser in helping patients feel comfortable in seeking help from others, or the critical "whole family" approach of pediatric practice. It does, however, force us to move beyond the easy and exclusive reliance on the medical community to meet the needs of all persons living in families with HIV.

Defining the Family as the Focal System

As recently as 1993, researchers noted that "most studies of the psychosocial implications of HIV disease have been focused on the individual . . . yet for every person infected with HIV, there is a family and social support system that will also be affected."[2] Studies have shown that families, broadly defined, provide most of the care given to infected family members.[3] A child as young as nine or ten may become responsible for care of the ill parent, or an adolescent sibling may assume surrogate parenting responsibilities for younger siblings. A grandmother or aunt may take the children of an ill parent into her home, or the child may pass through a number of foster family homes or more loosely defined family kinship arrangements. If a surviving parent has remarried or is living with another adult, the HIV-affected children may live in a reconstituted family, possibly with newly acquired siblings.

Authors of earlier chapters have argued for a broadened and more functionally based definition of *family*. Especially in the context of children affected by HIV, the notion of family must be broadened beyond parents and siblings to include the multigenerational extended family (grandparents, aunts, and uncles) and then to the chosen family network (godparents, family friends) as well. By expanding the notion of family we can build support for children based upon the much broader social, cultural, and caregiver networks that naturally surround them.

Importantly, in both extended and chosen families, all participants must be viewed as HIV affected. We know from the general clinical literature that when any family member undergoes dramatic disability or illness, whether acute or chronic, all members of the family are affected. With specific regard to HIV disease, "family members may display the same psychological symptoms as the infected person, ranging from fear, anger, agitation, and withdrawal to anxiety and depression."[4]

This broadened view of family has several implications for the provision of service. First, for the multigenerational family system to function well as a resource for the affected child, there are often issues between the infected adult and his or her parent that must be addressed before the grandparent can effectively "take on" parenting the uninfected grandchild.[5] These issues include unresolved dependency, guilt over earlier conflicts, anger over earlier rejections. Because repairing these relationships between parent and grandparent must occur before the infected parent dies, clinical support in the critical issue of *telling* may become essential. Second, the child's given or chosen caregivers will likely require clinical, emotional, and often financial support similar to that needed by the infected parent or parents. This need may present a significant challenge to current providers of services, who are often trained to work with a single patient; they may not understand the cultural context of family systems and may therefore view the family network as confusing or chaotic. Finally, at a time in which insufficient resources are directed at meeting the needs of affected children, expanding the definition of need further stresses the service system.

Despite these challenges, families will continue to provide the context for much of the care and support given to children affected by HIV. As policymakers and providers, we must devise effective ways of reaching families with the supports necessary for children to survive this epidemic.

Working from a Developmental Understanding of Children's Needs

All children progress through a series of general developmental periods and face a number of predictable tasks, as described in Chapter 3. For the young child, cognitive, language, and emotional development generally occurs within the circle of immediate family or consistent caregivers, and parental and sibling relationships are extremely important. As children become preschoolers, their social world generally expands to include other youngsters in play environments. Starting school represents a major transition, as children enter the teachers' world, and the circle of peer acquaintances expands. During this period, children make great cognitive and social gains and begin to develop their expressive and physical competencies through the arts and sports. By the end of elementary school, peer relationships have grown in impact and import, and the children face the transition to intermediate school, where their circle of friends and educational adults (teachers, coaches, activity leaders) expands again. Adolescence marks yet another transition, physiologically with maturation of the body and the emergence of sexuality, and cognitively as children become able to engage in more abstract thinking. School pressures increase, some youths become employed, and the struggle between dependence upon and independence from family and friends reaches a new intensity.

While the pacing of children through these periods of growth and change may vary according to individual, cultural, and environmental circumstances (including living with HIV disease), all children have a common set of basic needs:

- Essential physical services: a safe place to live, food, and clothing.
- At least one nurturing, consistent older person (generally a parent) in whom to trust.
- Success in primary environments: school/child care, peer groups, recreation/sports/play, and work.
- Success in personal communication through spoken or written language and/or artistic or physical expression.
- A group to belong to.
- Safe physical outlets for energy.
- Someone or something else to be responsible for and take care of.

To varying extents, these basic developmental needs may conflict with responsibilities or worries associated with being a child in a family with HIV disease. For example, the very young child needs a strong positive physical relationship with a consistent adult, but if that adult is bedridden, fatigued, or repeatedly hospitalized with an AIDS-related illness, contact and bonding will be negatively influenced. The eight- or nine-year-old child affected by HIV may want to be with friends playing soccer or streetball but may be afraid or unable to leave an ill parent. Equally likely, the preadolescent may miss school while caring for the infected parent and be unable to explain the absences to the teacher. The teenage sibling who needs to be with male and female peers at school and social events may also be functioning as the surrogate parent, requiring a constant presence at home.

Responsive social systems working with children in families with HIV must find ways to identify these fundamental conflicts and create opportunities for children to be children. This responsibility may fall on the educational, juvenile justice, recreational, and faith communities because children's early behavioral indications of family disruption due to HIV disease may first be evident there.

Resilience: Characteristics of the Child, the Family, and External Social Support

The expanding body of clinical and developmental literature on resilience helps us to understand why some children, facing significant ongoing stress and trauma, are apparently able to experience social and cognitive competence and school success.[6] Three main factors appear to contribute to the resilience of such children: the manner in which the child approaches challenges; the nature of the child's experience within the family; and the nature of external supports that exist for the child and family.

Each of these domains—the child, the family, and supports beyond the family—operates in interaction with the others in the context of the child's and family's culture, the child's developmental level, and the relative well-being of the parent. Importantly, resilience develops not from a life absent of crisis but in response to problems tackled at a time and in a way that build the individual's successful coping and problem-solving repertoire.[7]

Characteristics of the child. Cognitive and social characteristics (both innate and learned) contributing to the capacity of the resilient child to rebound from trauma and extreme stressors appear to include:

- *An active orientation toward problems:* The resilient child approaches problems with the view that they can be solved, then initiates action.
- *Persistence in problem-solving activities:* The resilient child makes repeated attempts at problem resolution based on the likelihood of success and feedback from each attempt.
- *A range of strategies to respond to problems:* Rather than limiting action to one strategy or approach, the resilient child employs a variety of intellectual and social strategies to solve a problem and is flexible in moving from one to another based on ongoing information.
- *A broad range of interests and goals:* The resilient child approaches the world with a strong curiosity about things, people, and ideas.
- *Social adeptness:* Resilient children are skilled at using their social world, including peers and adults, to provide critical support, and they are readily able to elicit positive responses from others, especially adults.

Family structure and relationships. Family characteristics that contribute to the resilience of children include:

- More, rather than less, physical and psychological space for family members.
- A strong bond between the child and the primary caretaker or caretakers during infancy.
- Empathetic understanding and support of the child as a unique being.
- A consistent relationship between the child and at least one parent, characterized by high levels of warmth and the absence of severe criticism.
- Good parental supervision, with clear rules and balanced discipline.
- Flexibility in dealing with situations in which the child's agenda and the parent's agenda do not agree.
- Capacity of the parent to contain parent-child problems to the immediate situation rather than allowing them to influence subsequent interaction.
- Cohesiveness of family members.
- In the absence of the parent, an older sibling or other adult with whom the child can bond as a caregiver and confidant.

Role of external support. The third factor in the resilience triad involves personal contact and connections with supportive persons and networks beyond the family. These persons and networks, present in times of celebration and need, provide financial, physical, emotional, social, and spiritual support.[8] Although these natural networks generally include the extended family, close neighbors and friends, and other persons and groups, specific membership will vary across cultural groups and will differ for children and adults as well. For children, external support means access to caring adults in whom to trust and safe places to expend energies and express emotions. It can also mean phone contacts and even anonymous conversations on electronic bulletin boards. Support networks for children often include same-age friends, older friends, religious leaders and church organizations, and, in some cases, teachers and coaches. Sources of support for adults include immediate and extended family members, broader networks of friends, gatherings at religious activities, and even phone access to other adults.[9]

A summary note on the resilience model. Taken together, these characteristics of the child and family, coupled with the presence of a network of social supports, appear to result in a pattern of positive adaptation for children of divorced, alcoholic, or mentally ill parents, children living through wars and disasters, and children living in extreme socioeconomic disadvantage. In all of these groups of children, the critical challenge in fostering resilience appears to involve increasing strengths in one domain when another is stressed.

Research on childhood resilience has critical applicability for the development of responsive support systems for HIV-affected children. First, it forces us to seek out particular strengthening experiences for them. These include promoting at each phase of development a child's empowered and successful interaction with the world around him or her, as well as assuring the presence of a consistent, nurturing adult in the child's life. Second, the research confirms that the presence or absence of effective support systems plays a critical role in the development of resilience. Especially when families are under extreme stress, it is in these positive support networks that children find rewards and a sense of belonging. If belonging is not found in safe environments characterized by the constructive use of energy and expression, it will be sought in other, more dangerous contexts, including early sexual encounters, drug and alcohol use, and gang participation. Third and perhaps most important, by applying the principles of resilience, caring adults and professionals in these external environments can structure their interactions with children and families to maximize the likelihood of positive child development and successful coping skills.

The words and drawings of children included at various points in this volume speak eloquently of the power of resilience in the face of AIDS. Perhaps most compelling is the story "My Life," reproduced in full later in this volume. It was written by a fifteen-year-old boy, a straight-A student in school, whose parents have both died of AIDS. He lives with his two younger siblings in the home of his aunt, who has four other children. He is seeking a job to help with household finances. The excerpt that follows is presented exactly as written:

> My life has been good. For the first 10 years I had a loving mother and my family lived very close to each other. My mother was a very good mother and I new that she loved us very much. . . . [On my 12th birthday] she said I think your old enough and I'm going to tell you what was wrong. . . . I was stuned because I could not beleive that my mother was going to die the only person that nurised me when I was sick and she told me and my brothers and sisters that if we wanted to make her happy was to stay in school and get an education and she will be the happiest mother in the world. I started crying and she hugged me and said that every thing would be all right because aunty would be there for us and that she will not let anything happen to us. . . . I said all right I will try to be strong for my brother and sisters. . . . Now I'm 14 going on 15 and me my brother and sister is living with our aunt and every thing is all right for us.
> Signed: S.O.S.—Some One Special.

Cultural and Religious Contributions and Diversity

Perhaps the broadest networks that can exist around children and families are those based upon their cultural and religious heritage. As Nora Groce pointed out in Chapter 6, both culture and religious experience help to frame expectations about family roles and obligations, responses to crises and death, and ways of celebrating life and success. Often, one is best understood within the context of the other, though each has the capacity to build quite a different system of support around, and on behalf of, families.

Though we may describe both culture and religious experience as unitary constructs, underlying each is a richly diverse set of views, values, and constructions of reality specific to both heritage and geography. Americans from Puerto Rico, Colombia, or Mexico may have been similarly described as "Latino" or "Hispanic," yet each culture has its own specific characteristics, and uninformed or simplistic generalizations can lead to significant clinical and social errors. Similarly, Roman Catholic Americans from Puerto Rico, Colombia, or Ireland share a religious orientation, but where culture and religion intersect, each group is significantly different from the others.

Educators and human service professionals talk regularly about the need to celebrate children's cultural heritage. However, service delivery is not generally based on an understanding of how cultural diversity affects the ways that families work, the ways that children and families think about problems, and the nature of their external support systems. Nor do the human services regularly communicate with families in the language of their culture, even if it is literally the only language the families speak. Yet such cultural and linguistic sensitivity is critical when working with families from diverse backgrounds if trust is to be established and access granted. With specific regard to services for families living with HIV, such problems are exacerbated by the failure or inability of many of the formal helping systems to employ a sufficiently multicultural work force.

Equally important for families living with HIV disease, where issues of death and dying cannot be avoided, is the role of the family's spiritual community, a critical base of potential social support or recrimination. Some faith communities view AIDS as punishment for moral failures and offer only the prospect of suffering in this life and the next. Others view persons with AIDS with the compassion accorded anyone with a terminal disease.[10] For families who are living with HIV and have strong ties to organized religions, views expressed by the clergy can offer both spiritual and social support, or they can magnify the secrecy and isolation that families already feel. For families who experience a more private spirituality, the presence of a personal belief system can assist in the development of positive coping skills.[11]

Marva's story, presented at the end of this volume, speaks eloquently to the importance and power of spirituality. Marva's two sons have HIV disease, her daughter-in-law has died of AIDS, and she is helping to care for her eight grandchildren. Marva says, "You know, we have an old saying that God doesn't put on us anymore than we can bear. You learn that you can *take a lot* if you have to—that you don't have to fold up and give up." She continues: "There's life after HIV. I thought it was the end of the world, but it's not. Life goes on. I didn't think that way for a long time. . . . I think I must have begged God all day long, 'Please don't take my child,' . . . [but] I changed my prayer. . . . 'Everyday that you let me have him, I'll be thankful.' Everyday, because this is the day that the Lord has made, and whatever day it is, I'll be grateful. . . . I thanked him for everyday that he let me have him. So that's the way that I get through things."

Understanding the contribution of cultural and religious beliefs and developing respect for their diversity is critical if we are to meet the needs of children and families living with HIV. Supportive members of these communities must be acknowledged as essential people in the lives of HIV-affected families, included as legitimate caregivers, and assisted as part of the extended family network.

Fitting Services to the Needs of Children

There is a substantial literature on the need to reform traditional human service programs.[12] Fragmented programs, the absence of collaboration among providers, gaps in funding, difficulty in gaining access to existing services (whether because of scheduling rigidity, transportation inadequacy, and/or linguistic insensitivity) are well documented. It is clear that many children and families in the greatest need find it difficult if not impossible to navigate the complex web of human services. For some children and some needs, there is simply no service or appropriate help available. Across geography and type of service agency, children and families are routinely fit into existing structures rather than the reverse.

Redefining service delivery for children affected by HIV disease has several requirements. First, natural social networks—including extended families, schools, peers, and neighborhood-based organizations—must be seen as the first line of support for affected children. For it is within special relationships in these normative settings that affected children may feel secure enough to give voice to their feelings, fears, and questions. Although people within these networks will vary by choice of the child and family, they must be supported—emotionally and financially—and included, as appropriate, in the planning that goes on to meet the needs of these children. Second, community-based family support organizations and mental health agencies, willing to provide services within the home, may become the most essential clinical supports for both children and families. Third, both family support and mental health resources need to be available to families and their children before problems—including planning who will care for children after death of the parent—reach crisis levels. Fourth, clinicians must be trained and comfortable in working with the multigenerational family systems of both the infected family and the child's chosen family (including foster and adoptive families arranged for through the child welfare system). Fifth, when affected children have no appropriate family resource available to them, therapeutically designed options for group living and supported transitional living must be made available. Finally, when service needs cross categorical boundaries, providers must agree on which agent will have primary case management responsibility and how services will be integrated into the lifespace of the family and the children.

Challenges to Agents of Support and Service

That "it takes a village to raise a child" has become a widely accepted call to action among reform-oriented child advocates, scholars, and social service providers.[13] This old African maxim has a profoundly simple meaning: many members of a community must cooperate in ensuring that its children receive the support and positive growth opportunities that they require. Nowhere is this guidance more urgently appropriate than for children living through AIDS. Yet nowhere may it be more difficult to accomplish.

Change Over Time: A Complicating Dimension

To identify the challenges implicit in "becoming a village," we must understand the changes *over time* within the family living with HIV. The first and most obvious context of change is the ten- to twelve-year course of the disease itself for infected parents. Though much of its symptomology, illness, and physical decline occur over the final two to three years of the parent's life, diagnosis will likely have come much earlier, initiating all of the psychological and social effects on the family that have been described in other chapters. As the disease progresses, the economic and housing situations of the family may be affected as well.

"Matthew," in his story presented later in this volume, describes just this chain of events. Matthew was director of an AIDS residence. He is HIV infected and is the father of a five-year-old uninfected son. He explains: "If I was to get sick tomorrow, just as any of my clients who have full-blown AIDS, one by one I lose things. I lose my job, because I can't do it anymore. I lose my income because I'm not working. I lose my insurance. I lose my home and my son loses his home with me. . . . He starts to lose the support of me, as his father. I start becoming too weak to give him the things he needs from a father, and little by little I end up with nothing. So, at the end of this chain of events, you have Matthew with basically nothing [and you] have his five year old son witnessing this whole, awful, terrible dilemma and being traumatized by it." To address these issues, the helping process must vary over time, with an early and continuing emphasis on psychological support and the inclusion of direct physical and financial assistance later in the course of the disease.

In addition to living with a parent who is infected with HIV, well children in the family may also have one or more siblings who are infected. This adds yet another level of complexity to family dynamics. Children infected with HIV appear to follow one of two courses: the young child becomes very ill and dies within the first two years, or the infected child lives into adolescence. In the first case, there will be significantly more medical involvement in the family early on, directed at efforts to treat and save the life of the young child. In the second case, support will more often be directed at helping the infected child, and his uninfected siblings, learn to live with chronic illness.

Another context for change is the natural developmental progress of the uninfected child over this same period. As noted earlier, the particular phase of cognitive development for a given child will help determine how that child understands both the parent's illness and the attempts of others to give assistance. In many families living with HIV, there are several children, often representing a broad age range and thereby complicating the helping situation even further. The nature of the child's social relationships changes as well over this period, evolving from a reliance on direct family members to a predominant role for friends and outside adults. As the nature of the child's primary relationships changes, his or her willingness to seek and accept help from the community will change as well. This natural course of developing social relationships becomes even more significant if the family experiences several physical relocations, with accompanying changes in schools, teachers and coaches, friends, and neighborhood groups.

Similarly, the child's developmental stage and experience may influence who becomes the new caregiver and how that relationship functions over time. A family is almost always sought for young children who become orphaned or whose own parents become unable to provide safe care. However, older children who survive AIDS in their families may be unable or unwilling to accept integration into a new family context, whether within their own biological family or the foster care system, and placement with similarly aged children in a therapeutic group residence may provide for better outcomes. Even for children who are placed successfully with a new family while young, adolescence may bring dramatic changes in behavior related to earlier loss, prompting either short- or long-term placement within a treatment-oriented group setting.

Finally, if—as is often the case today—affected children in a family initially pass into the care of a grandparent or an aunt, we must understand changes over time in that caregiver's need for economic, emotional, and physical resources. Grandparents may be living on a retirement income, may have moved to smaller quarters, and may be struggling with ill health or disability themselves. With the introduction of children into the home, these challenges will increase rather than decrease over time. Extending assistance to the second family over the period of that family's care of the affected child or children, especially if the second family consists of an older adult with limited resources, may involve different support than was available for the infected parent.

The Helping Systems

Historically, child welfare, education, mental health, and legal services have been charged with protecting children and meeting their developmental needs. One would therefore expect to see these systems involved on some level with children affected by HIV disease. Yet these systems are already the least-well-funded and most beleaguered elements of our governmental safety net for children and families. The balance of this section briefly examines challenges specific to each of these traditional children's services. These challenges must be addressed if we are to create a developmentally appropriate "village" around children and families living with HIV disease. It also suggests an extended role for other community organizations as supports to children and their families throughout the course of the disease.

Challenges to Child Welfare Services

In this country, the child welfare system exists to secure a safe place for children to receive developmentally and culturally appropriate care when their parents or other family members cannot provide such care. The child welfare system's initial response to the crisis of AIDS in families focused on finding residences for infants and young children infected with HIV. To meet this need, the child welfare professionals recruited new groups of specialized foster parents, educated these parents and staff members about HIV disease, and provided access to a network of services for the infected child and foster family. In addition to foster homes, transitional residences were developed where groups of these children (called "boarder babies") could live until they could be matched with one of the specially trained foster families.[14] Having met the immediate needs of these infants, the child welfare system finds itself confronted by a new set of challenges in light of increasing knowledge about the course of HIV disease.

The door to service. Many families enter the child welfare system through the door to protective services, after allegations of neglect or abuse. In such instances, a child believed to be at imminent risk of injury may be involuntarily removed from the home and placed in foster care. If the child is not removed, the child protective services worker may become a constant presence in the home and lives of the family. From the perspective of the child protective system, such "intrusiveness" and the threat of removing the child are necessary means of keeping children alive and safe. From the perspective of a family living with HIV disease, however, the perceived risk of losing custody of its children "to the state" is reason enough to avoid voluntary contact with the child welfare system.

Thus one challenge to the child welfare system is to establish or enhance a process or structure—separate and distinct from child protective services—through which families can request and receive home-based services on a truly voluntary basis. Agents of these voluntary child welfare services may be employees of the state, or they may work for community organizations on contract to assist families in meeting the varied needs of their children. However, it is critical for state and municipal child welfare employees—and families—to understand and respect this real distinction between child protective services and child welfare services. Specialized training is required to support workers in each of these related functions. Insofar as the functions are truly separate and parents are able to perceive their differences, families living with HIV may seek the custody and placement planning help that they now so often avoid. As we have seen in earlier chapters, because financial support is so often tied to the receipt of formal child welfare services, it is imperative that parents become able to request assistance from this system.

Family preservation and support services. As described more fully in Chapter 9, the 1993 federal Family Preservation and Support Services Act mandates that states make available an array of home-based services, designed to support families and to enable them to remain intact. These services, generally directed in practice toward preservation of biological families, may be provided by the child welfare agency itself or through contract with a community service organization. Component services may include programs for home health care, respite care, child care, crisis intervention, and mental health, as well as transportation and even short-term financial support. Families living with HIV disease may find these services accessible only through the child welfare agency.

Although families living with HIV may qualify for both family preservation and family support services, there are important differences in how each is intended to function. Family preservation services are generally initiated for a family in which a child is at imminent risk of placement due to abuse or neglect. Services are relatively short in duration but may be provided within the family around the clock. The delivery of family preservation services can be very costly because of their intensity and the utilization of highly trained clinical professionals. Family support services are less expensive, utilizing resources in the community to help empower families to resolve their own problems. Importantly, family support services are generally made available before a family reaches a crisis stage.[15]

As is clear from this and other chapters, elements of both programs are needed by families living with HIV. Yet child welfare administrators, faced with insufficient services for children who are abused or at risk of abuse, may argue that families living with HIV disease are not at sufficient risk to warrant access to either or both programs. The tragedy of such a policy decision is predictable: failure to support children and families during the course of this disease will likely result in significant—and more costly—mental health problems later in the children's development. The challenge to the child welfare system becomes one of creating a sufficiently large service base so that no families who are eligible for these federally mandated services are denied access to them.

The problem of placement. As we have repeatedly seen throughout this volume, the issues of custody and placement of HIV-affected children are of paramount importance in families where the sole parent or both parents are dying. Though not generally the parent's placement resource of choice, the child welfare system will be involved with many children affected by AIDS.

There are several challenges to effective service delivery for these children. First, the child welfare system must establish a means of planning with the family for a nurturing environment for its children when it is clear that the given family will be unable to secure an appropriate setting or when the chosen family requires access to clinical or financial support for a period of time. Second, the system must make sound clinical recommendations about placement of HIV-affected children with a family versus placement in a therapeutic group setting. Third, the system must be open to a family's choice of kinship placement and must develop means to support these chosen families, both clinically and at financial rates equivalent to those paid to foster parents.[16] Fourth, the child welfare system must overcome its historic inability to develop sufficient permanent placements for children of color, for the growing number of HIV-affected children will not make this problem any easier. Regulations limiting the number of children placed with one foster family may need to be relaxed for children coming from AIDS-affected families in order to keep the siblings together as a family unit. Finally, a system of transitional, voluntary placement needs to be developed. Children living in families with AIDS need to be able to move easily to an appropriate placement in their home community while the parent is hospitalized, allowing for continuity in the child's peer group and educational environment, and then to return home when the parent again is able to care for the child.

Children who serorevert. Infants born to women infected by HIV will test HIV positive at birth because they carry maternal antibody. Though currently only about 25 percent of these infants are actually infected, obtaining a definitive diagnosis has until recently taken some time. Some of these children, often those of substance abusing women unable to reliably care for them, come into the foster care system. As noted earlier, such children frequently are served as part of a specialized child welfare caseload. Characteristics of service delivery generally include higher payment rates for the foster family, smaller caseloads for the worker, and special training for both.[17] This system has worked well in providing a base of highly qualified homes for HIV-antibody–positive children. However, the well-documented reversion to HIV-negative status of many of these children, coupled with new capacity to make an early and definite diagnosis, raises a number of challenges for policymakers.

Because about 75 percent of these children are not actually HIV infected and an early diagnosis is now possible, should their care be reimbursed at a significantly higher rate than that of other children, including siblings affected by AIDS, who are also in need of foster or adoptive homes? When these children serorevert, should they be moved to nonspecialized programs or homes, generally at a lower foster care rate of reimbursement, or returned to a placement with their noninfected siblings in a single home, thus recreating the biological sibling family? What happens if the foster family falls in love with the parentless child, who is now affected but uninfected? Is adoption encouraged? If an adoption is consummated, will the child and the new family continue to be eligible for support services through the child welfare agency?

As the child welfare community debates these difficult questions, the principles of resilience must be applied as guidance in the placement of each individual child. Family ties need to be continued when possible. Siblings should not be denied the opportunity to grow up together when that is clinically viable. A consistent, nurturing caregiver needs to be identified and the relationship with this person established. Cultural bonds need to be respected, but children must not be allowed to languish in foster care.

Planning and services integration. As must be clear at this point, no single agency will be able to meet the complex needs of all children and families living with HIV. Similarly, any given family will need various types of supports over the course of the disease. The need for a multidisciplinary and multiagency approach may pose a challenge to the child welfare system, which sees itself as the primary agent of support for children at risk. Other challenges also exist for child welfare, including the need for specialized training for workers, effective information sharing within families and across helping agencies, and the need for a seamless, coherent case management system.

The child welfare system nationally is faced with an enormous task even before it begins to address the needs of these children. According to recent estimates, 400,000 children are in foster care, with more than half a million expected by 1995.[18] The significant number of children who will require both in-home support and a second family will further tax an overburdened and underfunded system.[19]

Challenges to the Educational System

With the possible exception of television viewing, schools occupy the single greatest block of children's time from the age of five or six through at least early adolescence. Schools tend to the cognitive, language, social, emotional, and physical growth of children and provide opportunities for personal expression through the arts and for physical skill development through sports. Schools also provide entry to the world of work and, until recently, were generally viewed as safe places to gather with peers and friends. The educational experiences of children in school in all of these contexts—classroom learning, social activities, the introduction to work, sports, and artistic expression—offer students the opportunity for success so essential to resilience.

As both Shelley Geballe and Jan Hudis have argued earlier, schools have a vital role to play in the prevention of AIDS and as an early source of support for children in HIV-affected families. All states have a mandate for schools to provide students with health education, and some school districts have established health clinics within middle and high schools.[20] All schools have a mandate to identify students with special needs, and some schools offer teachers training in recognizing behavioral symptoms of family crisis. Some schools provide students with access to mental health services, including bereavement counseling. All schools speak of the importance of parental involvement in the education of their children, and many districts make school resources available to parents as well.[21] The literature on resilience tells us that the efforts of schools to meet the needs of children buffeted by family stress, illness, and dysfunction must increase as the family's resources dwindle. Access to all of these types of school-based services are critical for children living in families with HIV disease.

There are, however, several important challenges facing school systems if they are to become members of the HIV-affected child's village. Schools must serve as an early warning system for children struggling through life with HIV disease in their families, yet current confidentiality statutes prohibit disclosure of the HIV status of parents, even when such disclosure would assist staff to understand and respond to the needs of children for specialized support. Schools also must serve as a source of mentors and positive adult role models and as a link with other community resources for both children and families. To do so, teachers and administrators must receive training about HIV disease and its impact on children and families. Such training will address their concerns about the communicability of the disease, challenge any prejudice they may have and be communicating to students and families, and enable them to better meet the predictable needs of these children. Finally, urban school systems, where most children currently affected by HIV receive their education, are notoriously underfunded, undermaintained, and understaffed. In some of these districts, students can be absent for days or months without effective follow-up. Textbooks used in some districts predate the appearance of HIV disease in 1981. Some schools must choose between hiring teaching or security staff. It is difficult to imagine such environments undertaking yet another service for children and youths—comprehensive AIDS-specific health education, school-based health and mental health services—without additional resources for staffing and training. Similarly, sports activities offer children a positive, structured outlet for physical energy, arts activities enable children to develop new means of expression, and both offer children positive adult role models, yet both sports and the arts are routinely reduced or eliminated when school budgets are tight. Such funding must be restored.

Challenges to Mental Health Systems

Earlier chapters bear witness to the immense psychological journeys awaiting children and families living with HIV as they struggle with the trauma of multiple death, social stigma, and personal silence. It is instructive, at this point, to speculate on the specific journeys which face Charlie and Joey, whom we met at the beginning of this chapter. From his writing, we know that Joey will live each available moment, doing psychological battle with the virus that infects him. He will speak out, and he will garner support from those around him. From Charlie's silence, we suspect that he will attempt to move on without confronting the anger and pain that reside deep within him. Though Charlie chooses not to voice them, these feelings will remain, and we can predict that at some point, perhaps at the death of his brother, Charlie will need—perhaps even want—psychological help.

Many of the previous chapters have presented a strong case for access to mental health services for children and families affected by HIV—crisis intervention services, bereavement counseling, multigenerational family therapy, and support groups for children and for both given and chosen families. The authors have properly argued that such mental health services should reflect the linguistic and cultural preferences of a family, be appropriate to the stage of illness within the family and to the developmental level of the children, and be available to families at convenient times and in accessible locations.

Developing responsive, appropriate, and accessible mental health services for HIV-affected children and their families requires that several challenges be addressed. Perhaps most significant is the inadequacy of existing mental health services for children in general and for adolescents in particular. In some communities, mental health services are available only to those in acute psychological crisis; in others, services are not accessible unless a family has private health insurance. Frequently, services are offered only in English by Anglo-American professionals, and recurrent problems in sharing information and authority may restrict the effectiveness of a cross-agency team approach.

A second and more subtle challenge facing the mental health system is the ongoing tension between professionals who emphasize the need to work with individual patients and those who believe that the entire family constitutes the necessary unit for effective intervention. There is also a recurrent tension between clinical disciplines that stress the need for long-term psychotherapy and those that promote short-term interventions geared toward the development of coping skills. Families and children living with HIV need access to a range of therapeutic models, delivered by clinicians who understand that building trust within these families may take time and who are willing to work with family members in their homes.

Finally, there is the challenge for mental health professionals to recognize the extraordinary fragility that children and their families develop after repeated experiences with physical suffering, social stigma, and multiple deaths. HIV disease is not a single sudden illness in which one day you are vigorous and the next day you are gone but rather a progressively more visible process that brings physical wasting, dementia, and a need for medication and support apparatus. There is no way for a child to live in a family with AIDS, even if it is not *named,* and fail to see frightening physical changes in the parent the child loves and believes to be invincible. AIDS is not cancer, which inspires communities to rally around a child and a family where a parent is terminally ill. There are no bake sales or car washes to raise money for the AIDS family, no constant press of neighbors and acquaintances bringing food and comfort. AIDS is not only one parent dying but often the second parent too, as well as uncles, aunts, cousins, and siblings. There is not a single period of mourning but rather overlapping cycles of grief.

HIV disease demands much from families. It also demands much from the mental health professionals who carry the silent burden of this epidemic on their shoulders as well. Care for these caregivers is perhaps the mental health system's least recognized challenge.[22]

Challenges to the Legal Community

As seen in Chapter 9, the legal community has a significant role to play in addressing the needs of children affected by HIV disease, through legislation and legal services to combat prejudice, provide options for the placement and custody of orphaned children, and facilitate the delivery of health services to children.

There are important challenges as well. First, the legal community must provide adequate and timely representation of and for children. Representation must be available to parents who are planning the legal transfer of custody of their children and for those children who will become wards of the state as their parents die. This effort will require adequate funding for courts to engage competent attorneys on behalf of children and indigent families. It will also require specialized training for counsel and judges about HIV, child development, the dynamics of family functioning, death and grieving, entitlement planning, and custody law.

A second challenge demands improvements in the processing of probate court home studies necessary to confirm changes in custody. A significant backlog of custody cases awaiting home study and disposition already exists within the probate court system. This situation will be exacerbated when large numbers of HIV-related custody cases are filed, forcing processing time to extend beyond what is reasonable for a child. A one-year-old who has spent six months awaiting finalization of a relative adoption has spent 50 percent of his or her life awaiting permanency. This challenge can be addressed with funding for additional probate judges and for additional staff to complete home studies in a more timely manner.

Finally, the juvenile justice system, as an arm of the legal community, will continue to receive children and youths whose problematic behaviors may have resulted, in part, from the psychological trauma of living with AIDS in their families. Juvenile detention and incarceration facilities are generally understaffed, underfunded, and underprogrammed; they are poor environments for the delivery of rehabilitative and mental health services. Significant diagnostic improvements, along with enhanced treatment opportunities, must be made available for HIV-affected children in these systems.

Challenges to Community Resources

For many children and families living in the United States, a broad range of community resources exists to provide children with activities before and after school and on weekends. Programs may be sponsored by the public schools, Girls and Boys Clubs, Scouts, community recreation departments, local arts organizations, religious groups, and such social service organizations as Lions Clubs. These programs often include both structured group activities and safe places to "hang out," and many are designed to promote leadership, community service, physical competence, and artistic expression.

For children living in families with HIV disease, such programs serve a critical function. All children and adults living in high-stress circumstances require a means of expressing their feelings in a context where that expression is likely to be welcomed and valued and where they are likely to feel some measure of success. As seen earlier in this volume, children's art provides an essential nonverbal means of expression. Sports and recreational activities can provide the opportunity to expend accumulated energy in a constructive manner. Besides serving a valuable quasi-clinical purpose, such activities allow children to "be children" at a time when family needs may be pressing them into adult responsibilities. Coaches and adult leaders of these activities may be willing to enter into a positive and nurturing relationship with these children when their adult role models lie ill and unable to interact with them. These varied normative and quasi-clinical functions available through community resources may satisfy many of the core needs of children and adolescents outlined earlier in this chapter.

There are challenges to be addressed, however, if community resources are to function well for children living with the traumas of HIV disease in their families. First, the resources must be available. As simple as that sounds, current economic realities for many communities have resulted in reductions in town- or city-sponsored recreational activities, and programs sponsored by private organizations are suffering from the current economic downturn as well. Second, resources must exist in settings where children need not fear for their safety. Finally, they must be places where children want to be.

Personal faith and spiritual understanding can play a significant and positive role in helping children and families cope with HIV disease.[23] For many children and families, the development of spiritual understanding comes through affiliation with a particular faith community, and all faith communities, regardless of their response to HIV disease, place a high value on the support of families. A community of faith can provide the social and material support needed to sustain and strengthen families through significant illness and may also function as an extended family for a family unit isolated from relatives. Some religious denominations have developed formal adoption programs for children affected by HIV.[24] Faith communities can also provide— through clergy, lay leaders and teachers—adults who can function as mentors and role models for children in desperate need of positive support.

The challenge for faith communities clearly concerns their theological and personal response to HIV disease among their parishioners. Messages of punishment subject families to further spiritual distress and social isolation. Silence on the part of the religious leaders may function in much the same way for those who are affected, as well as for those with HIV disease. The most inclusive message that a faith community can give is to acknowledge that when one member of the parish is infected with HIV, all members are affected.

Criteria for Program Design and Funding

Children affected by HIV have the same needs as all children: to be loved, to become competent, to have friends, to make a contribution, to be part of a community. But they have other needs as well. They need to be able to talk with someone about what is happening in their homes and in their lives. They need to be able to "make sense," at their own developmental level, of the deaths of the people who were supposed to protect them. They need permission to grieve. They need to know that there will be a place for them to be safe, tomorrow and next year.

The village around these children must include those who have a personal stake in their future, who speak their language, who understand their pain and can give them words for what they are feeling, who can provide opportunities for them to escape back into childhood, who can recognize their sacrifices, who can help them learn new roles and new rules. Members of the village will be different for different children and for the same children over time, but all members must have access to services that the child and family require and authority to negotiate on their behalf. If formal social service agencies are involved, a single case manager must represent them, and as a group they will need to determine which agency takes on this leadership role.

Just as there will be new challenges for children who have survived the death of their families, there will be new challenges for the people who work on behalf of those children. Community and provider representatives will need to work as a team, integrating their program offerings into the life cycles of the family. Natural supports from the community must be as welcome on the team as are the formal helping systems. The services offered must build on the strengths of the children and the family. Agency turf, rivalry, and unnecessary regulation must be left at the door. Information-sharing issues must be resolved at the outset. Members of both given and chosen families must be invited to participate and should expect to be supported as well. A family member may head the team. Training and staff development opportunities are essential as agencies adopt these new roles.

Perhaps the greatest challenge of this "helping team" will be to engage in relationships with the child and the family that foster resilience. Such relationships must invite children to have a voice, to participate in making choices, to become socially able to engage adult systems, to find alternative ways of meeting their goals, and to have multiple goals. Across the many people who will offer support, there must be at least one constant adult who has a personal, consistent, and nurturing relationship with each affected child. Finally, there must be recognition that the team and the new family will both be tested by the child until he or she is sure that the relationships are real and will last.

A Shorthand Test

The following six criteria provide a shorthand test for policymakers and professionals to evaluate funding and program decisions and a way for parents to evaluate whether a program is right for a child:

• Does the program stress surviving AIDS and identify the strengths of the child and family?
• Does the program accept the chosen family along with the given family as the unit of service?
• Does the program reflect the changing influence of the child's primary social environments: the family, the school and its teachers, peers, social groups, recreation, the workplace?
• Does the program promote resilience by fostering an active style of cognitive and social engagement on the part of the child and by providing a consistent, nurturing adult in whom the child can trust, as well as opportunities for valued expression and the likelihood of success?
• Does the program reflect sensitivity toward the child's culture, include representatives of the culture, and offer access to programs within the child's and family's local community?

• Is the program collaborative across services, integrated, and available to meet the needs of the family as they change over time?

These requirements constitute a rigorous test against which existing and new program services can be evaluated. Existing programs may not meet all of these criteria, but the decision to provide continued funding should take their compliance with these elements into account. New programs must be designed to satisfy all six criteria.

As the numbers of HIV-affected children in this country and in the world continue to increase, so will the intensity of their individual and collective needs. We will fail to meet these needs unless we reframe and then expand the supports and services available to them. Simply creating more of what we now have is not the answer.

Notes

1. Lopez, J. L., 1993, It's up to you, *Parabola* 18 (1): 68–71.

2. Bor, R., R. Miller, and E. Goldman, 1993, HIV/AIDS and the family: A review of research in the first decade, *Journal of Family Therapy* 15: 187–204. See also P. Wilson, 1993, HIV disease: Toward comprehensive services for families, in *The changing face of AIDS: Implications for social work practice*, ed. V. Lynch, G. Lloyd, and M. Fimbres, Westport, Conn.: Auburn House, 79–103; Bonuck, K. A., 1993, AIDS in families: Cultural, psychosocial, and functional impacts, *Social Work in Health Care*, 18 (2): 75–89.

3. Brown, M. A., and G. M. Powell-Cope, 1991, AIDS family caregiving: Transitions through uncertainty, *Nursing Research* 40 (6): 338–345.

4. Bor et al., see note 2 above.

5. Samperi, F., 1991, AIDS and survivorship: A three generational approach, available from the author at the Community Consultation Center, Henry Street Settlement, New York City; Samperi, F., 1993, AIDS and survivorship: A community-based mental health clinic's evolving response to the AIDS crisis, available from the author as above.

6. Rutter, M., 1993, Resilience: Some conceptual considerations, *Journal of Adolescent Health* 14 (8): 626–631; Luthar, S., and E. Zigler, 1991, Vulnerability and competence: A review of research on resilience in childhood, *American Journal of Orthopsychiatry* 61 (1): 6–22; Werner, R., and R. Smith, 1989, *Vulnerable but invincible*, New York: Adams Bannister Cox; Dunn, J., 1986, Stress, development, and family interaction. In *Depression in young people: Developmental and clinical perspectives*, ed. M. Rutter, C. Izard, and P. Read, New York: Guilford; Garmezy, N., 1993, Children in poverty: Resilience despite risk, *Psychiatry* 56: 127–136; Demos, E. V., 1989, Resiliency in infancy, in *The child in our times: Studies in the development of resiliency*, ed. T. Dugan and M. Rutter, 3–22, New York: Brunner/Mazel.

7. Rutter, see note 6 above.

8. Bronfenbrenner, U., 1979, *The ecology of human development: Experiments by nature and design*, Cambridge: Harvard University Press.

9. Luthar and Zigler, see note 6 above.

10. Doka, K. J., 1994, Suffer the little children: The child and spirituality in the AIDS crisis. In *AIDS and the new orphans: Coping with death*, ed. B. Dane and C. Levine, Westport, Conn.: Greenwood.

11. Nehring, W., K. Malm, and D. Harris, 1993, Family and living issues for HIV-infected

children, in *Women, children, and HIV/AIDS,* ed. F. Cohen and J. Durham, New York: Springer, 221–227.

12. Melaville, A. I., and M. J. Blank, 1991, *What it takes: Structuring interagency partnerships to connect children and families with comprehensive services,* Washington, D.C.: Education and Human Services Consortium.

13. H. Weiss, 1994, Building villages to raise our children, Presentation at the 1994 National Conference on Family Literacy, Louisville, Ky., April, 1994.

14. Anderson, G., 1990, *Courage to care,* Washington, D.C.: Child Welfare League of America.

15. See the *American Journal of Orthopsychiatry,* January 1989, 59 (1), an entire special issue of articles on family support services and the family support movement in the United States.

16. See Chapter 9 for a more detailed description of issues surrounding kinship care. See also H. Dubowitz, S. Feigelman, and S. Zuravin, 1993, A profile of kinship care, *Child Welfare* 62 (2): 153–169.

17. Child welfare professionals indicate formally that higher rates for specialized foster families to care for pediatric AIDS cases were established because of the levels of medical risk and the need for more intense care. Informally, child welfare employees indicate that higher rates were established as a recruitment and retention method.

18. Dubowitz et al., see note 16. See also Center for the Study of Social Policy, 1990, *The crisis in foster care,* Washington, D.C.: The Family Impact Seminar.

19. At this point, we do not know what proportion of these children are being served by or are otherwise already "known" to the child welfare system—because of referrals related to parental substance abuse, for example. Research is needed to assess the magnitude of the additional demand that will be placed on the system by the AIDS epidemic.

20. See Chapter 9 for a discussion of the legal arguments raised by opponents of school-based health clinics. See also R. A. Harold and N. B. Harold, 1993, School-based clinics: A response to the physical and mental health needs of adolescents, *Health and Social Work* 18 (1): 65–72.

21. A number of models for restructuring public schools, most notably Schools of the Twenty First Century, include family resource centers at the schools. These centers include day care for younger children, after-school care for students, and parenting and adult education for parents. See R. E. Behrman, 1992, School-linked services, *The Future of Children* 2 (1), Los Altos, Calif.: The David and Lucille Packard Foundation.

22. See Chapter 7 for a broader treatment of the need to care for caregivers, as well as the Agenda for Action in Chapter 12, which provides a list of policy and practice changes needed to effect support.

23. Mellins and Ehrhardt found, for example, that 86 percent of caregivers of children with HIV disease reported religion to be their most important and helpful coping strategy. Mellins, C. A., and A. A. Ehrhardt, 1994, Families affected by pediatric acquired immunodeficiency syndrome: Sources of stress and coping, *Journal of Developmental and Behavioral Pediatrics* 15 (3): S54–S60 (June supplement).

24. The Lutheran Church in Chicago, for example, runs a program called Second Families. A description of this program is included in the Resource Guide at the end of this volume.

Chapter 11

Today's Challenges, Tomorrow's Dilemmas
CAROL LEVINE

Only a few years ago there was scant public attention to the problems of children and adolescents living in families with AIDS and surviving the death of parents and siblings from the disease. As the chapters in this book demonstrate, that gap is being filled with new knowledge, new programs, and new, committed leaders. There are even some new, albeit inadequate, resources.

There is an urgent need to respond rapidly, even while a rigorous evaluation of service models goes on. A seriously ill mother needs legal help now in planning for her child's future. A grieving child needs emotional support now. An overburdened grandmother needs financial assistance and respite care now. Five years may ordinarily be a reasonable time for program development and evaluation, but for a ten-year-old it is the difference between childhood and adolescence—perhaps the difference between a chance for a secure future and serious trouble.

In such a crisis, it is inevitable and right that attention should be focused first on short-term solutions. Nevertheless, the future must also be considered. Given the current imperfect state of scientific and medical knowledge and the mixed results of prevention programs, there are no foreseeable prospects for ending the HIV epidemic. (Although some human viral diseases can be effectively treated or prevented, only smallpox has been eradicated.)

Moreover, according to the Centers for Disease Control and Prevention (CDC), current trends in AIDS case reporting project an even larger proportion of cases among women, racial and ethnic minorities, adolescents, injection drug users, and persons infected through heterosexual contact.[1] With the exception of a second wave of HIV among young gay men, all of the trends increase the probability that large numbers of orphaned children will survive.

Even a preliminary study suggesting that zidovudine (AZT) given to pregnant women and their newborns might reduce by as much as two-thirds the rate of maternal-child transmission carries with it the poignant reminder that the additional infants who escape HIV infection will still be orphaned.[2]

An epidemic, by definition, is a dynamic process. If there is one lesson that should have been learned from the first decade and a half of the HIV epidemic, it is that assumptions and programs need constant reevaluation to address changing conditions. Solutions that work for today's affected families may not be viable in the next generation. Controversial issues that are pushed aside today will arise tomorrow when there will be little time for sober reflection. The questions about the future are not limited to the impact of HIV disease on social systems, but in child welfare, as in so many other areas, the epidemic highlights the failures of existing systems. The primary goal of this chapter is to describe some future issues and begin to integrate them into current policy and programmatic discussions. Of necessity, the discussions must be somewhat speculative. Hard data are lacking in many crucial areas. First, though, a brief review of current recommendations is in order.

Recommendations for Immediate Action

Within the short time during which serious attention has been focused on the problem, a strong consensus has emerged about meeting the immediate needs of children and families. While there are disagreements about details and certainly a paucity of resources to implement programs, there is general agreement about the broad outlines. The following recommendations were developed in the course of The Orphan Project's work and are generally reflected in other chapters:[3]

- Mental health services, including bereavement counseling, should be enhanced and targeted to different ages, cultural backgrounds, service settings, and durations of service.
- Transitional services for youths and their new guardians should be created to provide an orderly move from AIDS-specific entitlements and services to more general programs.
- HIV-affected youths involved in family and juvenile court proceedings require proper evaluation and referral to appropriate community services, especially mental health services.
- Schools should be an important locus of child- and youth-centered services, HIV prevention programs, and staff training that focuses on confidentiality, affected children's special problems, and other family issues. Community and neighborhood programs targeting out-of-school youths are also essential because many of the most vulnerable youths do not attend school regularly.
- Supports for housing, including rent subsidies, should be created to keep existing families together and to promote the development and maintenance of new, stable family arrangements.

• Foster care agencies should develop flexible and supportive programs for voluntary placement of children during the parent's illness, return of the children during periods of good health, and, following the parent's death, continuing foster care with the same family, ideally leading to adoption.

• Agency regulations and federal and state laws should be revised to permit financial subsidies (to rent a larger apartment, for example) for low-income guardians who are not part of the foster care or pre-adoptive systems.

• New state laws (and federal laws that encourage or require states to enact such legislation) should be adopted to enable parents to appoint standby guardians. Such legislation should not jeopardize the guardian's eligibility for foster care or other subsidies.

Future Issues

Service Needs Outside Major Urban Centers

Programs that focus on orphaned youngsters and their families are concentrated in major urban centers. Although they in no way meet the needs of all the affected families in these cities, there exist at least some service models that can be replicated and adapted and some experienced workers to guide families and new workers. Of the estimated 82,000 to 125,000 children and adolescents in the United States and Puerto Rico who will have lost their mothers to AIDS by the year 2000, approximately 60 percent live in six cities: New York (an estimated 30,000), Newark (7,200), Miami (4,900), San Juan (4,200), Los Angeles (1,900), and Washington, D.C. (1,400). Less is known about how the remaining 40 percent are distributed.[4]

In its 1989 analysis of anonymous seroprevalence studies of newborns in thirty-five states that provide markers for the rates of HIV infection in pregnant women the CDC found the highest rates, not surprisingly, in urban health districts, primarily those in the Northeast and the South. The urban district that included Detroit was the highest in the Midwest, and the Las Vegas area was the highest in the West. More surprising and more important for future trends, high rates were also found in some nonurban districts, particularly in the South, where the highest nonurban rates were found in rural South Carolina.[5] Among southern states, seroprevalence has increased from 1.7 per thousand in 1989 to 2.0 per thousand in 1991.[6] A study of AIDS in rural North Carolina found a "two-way HIV freeway": residents who left rural areas and contracted HIV in cities return to their homes and contribute to a rise in infection among hometown sexual partners. Over two hundred women are included in the study, 60 percent of them mothers. There were nearly 2.5 children per mother, and the children's average age was 8.9 years.[7]

Special problems for AIDS-affected families in nonurban areas include: (*a*) the general paucity of AIDS services for parents and uninfected children; (*b*)

long distances to travel to services, and isolation from people in similar circumstances; (c) the potentially greater degree of difficulty in maintaining confidentiality in small communities; and (d) the stigma surrounding AIDS, which
may be more severe in areas where AIDS is less common. On the positive side
it may be easier for a savvy case manager or social worker on the scene to
coordinate locally based services, to create flexible arrangements, and to avoid
delays in starting services.

The Lost Generation of Grandmothers and Aunts

Although data are scarce, it appears that when a mother dies of AIDS, children most often go to live—at least at first—with a grandmother or aunt.
Sometimes this relative has already been taking care of the children. In a pilot
study examining the outcome in forty-three cases that were closed shortly
after the mother's death, the New York City Division of AIDS Services found
that 58 percent of the children went to live with grandmothers or aunts.[8] In
Chicago, twenty-one of seventy-two HIV-infected mothers who were interviewed about future plans indicated that they would like their mothers to take
the children; nine designated their sisters, and twenty-two designated other
relatives.[9] Twenty were not able to identify anyone, and only fourteen of the
total made legal arrangements for their chosen caregiver. It is impossible to
predict how many of these plans will succeed, nor do we know the factors
that will influence different placement choices. One study looking at infants
born to HIV-infected women in six regions concluded that maternal drug use
may be the most important factor determining whether a child lives with a
biologic parent. In all locations and for all racial and ethnic groups, a newborn
whose mother used intravenous drugs was more likely to be placed with
someone other than the mother.[10]

The phenomenon of skip-generation parenting—children being raised by
grandparents instead of parents—is not solely attributable to HIV disease. Use
of drugs, especially crack cocaine, has devastated many families. Grandmothers have taken over when their own children have been unable to take on
parenting responsibilities or when they have chosen to move their children to
a safer environment. This phenomenon has particularly affected African-
American communities. As of 1990, 12 percent of black children in the
United States were living with grandparents, compared with 5.7 percent of
Hispanic children and 3.6 percent of white children.[11] The percentage of black
children living with grandparents in some urban areas is significantly higher,
with estimates ranging from 20 percent in a Head Start population in Oak-
land, California, to 30 to 70 percent in parts of Detroit and New York.[12]

Women have traditionally taken on the role of family caregiving. Many of
the grandmothers and aunts who take over the care of children whose

mothers have died of AIDS have additional family caregiving responsibilities—for their own children, spouses, partners, elderly parents, or other relatives. Two general outcomes are predictable. First, some of these women, no matter how willing and devoted they are, will be unable to continue to bear the escalating burdens because of illness, emotional exhaustion, poverty, or the severity of the children's behavior or academic problems. In one study of black grandparents, health problems such as diabetes, hypertension, back ailments, and low energy were often ignored because the health needs of the children took priority. Some of the grandparents viewed illness and death as their only escape from their burdens.[13] One grandmother described how she felt when she was faced with the responsibility of raising three HIV-infected grandchildren: "I was only 51, but I saw myself as a woman with no future."[14] Second, there will be no new generation of grandmothers to take the place of this generation—the lost generation of daughters will become a lost generation of grandmothers. For children, this vacuum represents a serious break in family continuity, which is already fragile in many cases. For the child welfare system, the shortage of grandmothers will mean increased pressure—possibly within five to ten years—on such alternatives to family placements as foster or congregate care.

The Impact on Adolescents and Young Adults

Skip-generation parenting has another facet: the younger generation may also be pressed to take on caregiving responsibilities out of the normal sequence of family life. The number of young adults (18 years and older) in the United States whose mothers die of HIV-related causes will reach 35,000 by 1995 and 64,000 through the year 2000.[15] While there are no data on the extent of the practice, and it is probably not typical, there are many anecdotal reports about teenagers and young adults taking over the care of younger brothers and sisters while the parent is ill and after the parent's death. Sometimes the young person became the parent's primary caregiver during the illness, and it is the parent's wish that the oldest child or oldest girl take over the care of the family.[16] This "parentification" of teenagers will have long-term consequences for their own futures, as well as for those of their younger siblings.[17] On the positive side, these adolescents may learn responsibility, effective coping mechanisms, and nurturing skills. However, they may also find themselves feeling overwhelmed and resentful that they have had to assume such a caregiving role, especially when their peers are in school or at work or simply having fun.

A possible model of service delivery for these adolescents is shared foster family care. Traditionally, this option places both parent and child in a foster home; young mothers take full responsibility for the children but are offered support and guidance by their foster parents.[18] Adolescents who become "parents" to their siblings could benefit from similar support. There are legal implications to these arrangements. A medical provider, for example, may be reluctant to allow a teenager to consent to elective surgery for a younger sibling. Sometimes an older person can be named as co-guardian if the law in the state permits a co-guardian arrangement and a lawyer is available to help formalize it.[19] In any case, the system must be able to assess the stability and security of these new family configurations and find ways to maintain viable households while still making educational and career opportunities available to the young person in charge. This is a formidable challenge.

An increasing percentage of young people are becoming infected through sexual transmission. Between 1992 and 1993, the largest increases in AIDS case reporting occurred among persons aged thirteen to nineteen years and twenty to twenty-four years; heterosexual transmission accounted for 22 percent of the infection in the younger group and 18 percent in the older group.[20] Some young HIV-infected women are also becoming pregnant. The study that showed a reduced rate of maternal-child HIV transmission in pregnant women taking AZT, for example, enrolled a fifteen-year-old girl as its youngest participant.[21] Such teenagers or young adults will face the same excruciating dilemmas about custody of their babies faced by older women—in some cases, their own relatives. The procedures, still new and exploratory, that guide women toward permanency planning will have to be refined in terms of adolescent development and diminished family resources.

Losses to Communities

The cumulative effect of the generational losses (added to the losses from drugs and violence) will have a serious impact on the social, cultural, and economic life of communities. Productive (or potentially productive) young adults will not be able to contribute to their families' and communities' income and welfare. Less tangibly, the continuous psychic assault of deaths upon deaths inhibits community healing. The reservoir of spiritual strength and resilience that still exists among individuals, families, and communities can be the source of positive actions, but the road will be hard. With a few exceptions so far, the use of the arts as catharsis that has characterized the gay community's response to the epidemic has not found a counterpart in minority communities.[22]

Institutional Child Care Settings

Orphanages—the very term conjures up images straight from Dickens: starving children abused by heartless masters. It is true that child care practices in some institutions in the United States and abroad, especially during the nineteenth century, seem punitive and rigid by contemporary standards. (Parenting practices of that earlier period would probably also fall short.) But some orphanages in the United States have provided good, even exceptional care. Several American social historians are elucidating the complex factors leading to the rise and fall of orphanages.[23] Children in institutions—first almshouses and then orphanages—were typically not orphans who had lost both parents. They often came, rather, from families where one parent was dead or ill, where there were so many children that the parents could not support them all, or where they were abused or neglected. If there was a stigma attached to being in an orphanage, it was often the stigma of poverty or, sometimes, of coming from an immigrant family.

Whatever the assessment of a particular institution at a particular time, the very suggestion that orphanages be revived guarantees controversy. The late Lois Forer, a family court judge in Philadelphia, saw the return of institutions as the only answer to the failure of families and foster care. "All institutions are not bad; all families are not good," she asserted in 1988.[24] Joyce Ladner, a professor of social work at Howard University, agrees. "What [children of dysfunctional parents] need is permanency, but the chances are that it will continue to be difficult to find adoptive families for these so-called high-risk youngsters," she says. "I advocate that we bring back the orphanage—not the huge, depersonalized warehouse of old, but small-scale caring institutions that can offer children, and their siblings, a place that they can count on to nurture them."[25] Some former residents of orphanages recall their experiences with fondness. At a reunion of graduates of the German Orphan Home in Washington, D.C., Elizabeth Harich Keiser said: "We had discipline, but it was good discipline. We were raised right, with good manners. We were happy there."[26]

On the other hand, the sentiment expressed most vigorously by President Theodore Roosevelt at the 1909 White House Conference on the Care of Dependent Children has survived to the present. In summing up the conference, Roosevelt said: "Home life is the highest and finest product of civilization. Children should not be deprived of it except for urgent and compelling reasons."[27] This conference was the beginning of the end of orphanages. The rise of professionalism of social work and the creation of a foster care alternative for dependent children, supported by psychoanalytically oriented research in the 1940s and thereafter, evolved into the prevailing doctrine that congregate care is always harmful to children.[28]

The primacy of family life has been stressed repeatedly in recent discussions. Believing that the family is the "most powerful and appropriate institution" for raising children, the National Commission on Family Foster Care, a joint project of the Child Welfare League of America and the National

Foster Parent Association, "flatly rejects the suggestion of some foster care critics that family foster care be supplemented by or replaced with orphanages." Although the commission acknowledges the overburdened and critical state of the foster care system, it criticizes those who would bring back orphanages as a solution: "Responding to the foster care crisis by dismantling foster care is a narrow approach that does not respect the diverse strengths and needs of children, youths, and families."[29] In this widely shared view, the emphasis should be on providing intensive services to preserve biologic families and on improving foster care, not on re-creating institutions.

Nevertheless, in some situations, congregate care is proving to be a useful, temporary option. Transition homes for HIV-infected babies have been successful in providing appropriate health care as well as emotional nurturing. These settings were created to offer an out-of-hospital environment for babies who had no homes until a longer-term placement can be arranged.[30]

Focusing on young children, however, avoids the harder issues. It is not as difficult to place infants and young children in families (whether in kinship care, foster care, or adoptive homes) as it is to place older children, particularly teenagers. If institutions are to be re-created, they will probably be to serve these harder-to-place youngsters. Also, some critics favor removing troubled youngsters from the dangerous environments of their communities and placing them in group settings where they can develop without the pressures of the drug trade and street violence. Group homes for teens already exist, with mixed results. Many orphaned adolescents are already in these placements, but there has been little attention to their special needs.

Views about removing youngsters from their homes and communities reflect different perspectives. William Bennett, former "drug czar" in the Bush administration, suggested that youths with drug-addicted parents and orphaned "teenagers up to the age of majority" should be placed in state- and community-run orphanages. He bluntly asserted that parents have failed. "We must save [children orphaned by drugs] by removing them from their biological family. . . . We should not assume that parents and family guardians are capable of providing for the physical, moral, and cognitive needs of the child."[31] By contrast, Thomas L. Webber, director of the Edwin Gould Academy, a public boarding school for foster care adolescents, stresses the importance of family members' participation in adolescents' lives and the creation of a "total learning community." The academy describes its living arrangements as "cottage or family style apartment" dwellings and, mindful of the negative views about institutions, insists that "no vestige of institutionalization will be allowed to creep into the cottage life."[32]

If youngsters who are removed from unhealthy environments return to them, they may be ill prepared to deal with the stresses. Yet if they do not return, their communities will have been deprived of some of the most effective agents of change—youngsters who have been afforded a better education and who have developed a stronger view of themselves and their ability to achieve productive goals. For the future, a rigorous, unemotional analysis of the appropriate role of congregate care—and the services that are needed to make it work in the interests of children—is essential.

Transracial Foster Care and Adoptions

Probably no single issue excites as much heated debate as the question of whether to place a child of one racial or ethnic background with a family of a different background. The current controversy primarily involves the placement of minority children in white families, because the vast majority of children available for adoption or foster care are African-American or Hispanic (as are the vast majority of children orphaned by AIDS), whereas the vast majority of families seeking children are white. In June 1993 in New York City, for example, 75 percent of the 17,826 children awaiting adoption were African-American. Nationally, African-American children comprise 40 percent of children awaiting adoption.[33]

The practice of transracial adoptions began in the 1950s and 1960s after the Korean War, when large numbers of Korean children were adopted by American families. In the 1960s and 1970s more than ten thousand African-American children were adopted by white families.[34] The National Association of Black Social Workers led the opposition to transracial adoption, calling it a "form of genocide." Its 1972 resolution, reaffirmed in 1985, states unequivocally: "Black children should be placed only with black families whether in foster care or adoption. Black children belong physically, psychologically and culturally in black families in order that they receive the total sense of themselves and develop a sound sense of their future. . . . Black children in white homes are cut off from the healthy development of themselves as black people."[35]

Similarly, the adoption of Native American children by white families was contested by tribal leaders. The 1978 Indian Child Welfare Act gave ultimate responsibility for child custody decisions, including adoption, to the child's tribe. As a result the incidence of adoption by white families from Native American groups is very low. A recent novel by Barbara Kingsolver describes the conflict arising from the adoption by a white mother of an abandoned and abused Cherokee girl and the tribe's subsequent efforts to regain custody.[36]

Because of the opposition of many (but not all) African-American and other minority leaders, transracial adoptions and foster care placements declined in the 1980s and 1990s. For example, of the 2,443 adoptions completed in New York City during the 1993 fiscal year, only 100 are estimated to have been transracial placements.[37] Now, however, the policy of same-race placement is itself being challenged. Elizabeth Bartholet, a law professor who adopted two Peruvian children, asserts: "There is extensive, unrefuted and overwhelmingly powerful evidence that the delays in permanent placement and the denials of such placement that result from current 'matching' policies do devastating damage to the children involved."[38] A review of the research on outcomes suggests that "transracial adoption is a viable means of providing stable homes for waiting children. It appears to produce children whose self-esteem is at least as high as that of nonadopted children and whose adjustment is highly satisfactory."[39]

Courts have held that absolute bans on transracial adoptions are unconstitutional under the equal protection clause of the United States Constitution. Neither are the respective races of the child and prospective parents factors that must be totally ignored in placement decisions. The current trend in the courts is to reject strong race-based preferences in placement laws, policies, or practices. Race is rather to be considered as one of many factors in determining the prospective adoptive parents' ability to meet all of a child's needs.[40]

The Multiethnic Placement Act (S. 1224), introduced by Sen. Howard Metzenbaum (D-Ohio), attempts to find a middle road. Senator Metzenbaum believes that "every child who is eligible for adoption has the right to be adopted by parents of the same race" and that "teaching a child self love and to embrace their racial and cultural heritage is more easily accomplished when parents and children are of the same race or ethnic group." Nevertheless, the bill prohibits state agencies or agencies receiving federal funds from totally prohibiting or unduly delaying transracial placements for either foster care or adoption. It attacks only the extreme versions of same-race policies, for example, the policy that allows white parents to foster black children but not to adopt them, even when a lengthy foster placement has engendered a strong bond. The act would presumably prohibit the practice in Connecticut of removing HIV-antibody–positive nonwhite infants from their original white foster families and placing them with the first available African-American or Latino family when the infants serorevert and thus prove to be uninfected. One similar case in New York is being challenged. In this instance, an agency is trying to remove a black child, who has seroreverted, from her Puerto Rican foster mother to be "reunited" in a black foster home with siblings whom she does not know.[41]

According to Randall Kennedy, a professor at Harvard Law School, Metzenbaum embraces "*moderate* racial matching." Kennedy opposes the bill and the very concept that race should be a factor in child placement. "Racial matching is a disastrous social policy both in how it affects children and in what it signals about our current attitudes regarding racial distinctions," he says. "Racial matching reinforces racialism. It strengthens the baleful notion that race is destiny. It buttresses the notion that people of different racial backgrounds really are different in some moral, unbridgeable, permanent sense."[42]

When strong beliefs are couched in terms of moral certainty, it is often difficult to analyze the situation clearly. What are the child's best interests in these cases? Embattled minority communities—whether African-American, Native American, Jewish, or any other—emphasize children as the future. Prospective adoptive parents and child advocates stress the future of the children. The reality, however, is more complex. A child has multiple identities— as a unique individual, as a family member, and as a member of an ethnic group, a religious group, a geographic community, and others.[43] Children's interests are best served by recognizing these overlapping identities and supporting solutions that lead to opportunity for full emotional, cognitive, and social development. Given the realities of American life, policies should neither ignore race nor place it above a child's total welfare.

Equity in Resource Allocation

By any standard of justice, it is unfair to pit one group of vulnerable children against another group. There can be no winners in such a contest. Advocacy for resources for children orphaned by the HIV epidemic must confront an uncomfortable question: Why do these children deserve special attention?

From the perspective of advocacy of children orphaned by AIDS, the death of a parent or sibling, especially a death from a stigmatized disease, makes a child particularly vulnerable. When a parent is absent or abuses drugs or alcohol, there is always a possibility—if only a fantasy—of a reunion and reconciliation. Death is final. One of the special needs occasioned by the death of a parent is bereavement counseling. Another need is for permanency planning.

From a child welfare perspective, there is no difference between the needs of the youngsters orphaned by HIV disease and their peers whose problems include substance abuse in the family, poverty, violence, and discrimination. Even the need for bereavement counseling applies to other children, including those who have lost family members and friends to other diseases or accidents or violence.

Yet from a pragmatic, short-term view, services must be targeted, and HIV disease is likely to be the driving force. For the long term, however, AIDS service organizations, especially those providing services to women and their children, should build alliances with child welfare organizations. In this way the special needs of the youngsters affected by HIV can be recognized and built into existing programs, and the problems that apply to the wider group of youngsters can be addressed in both settings. Wherever possible, it benefits all children to construct programs that meet generic as well as HIV-specific needs.

Beyond these programmatic and policy efforts, national leadership is important to focus attention on the inequitable distribution of resources that deprives American children of opportunities for health care, good educations, and secure and stable families. Despite rhetoric about being a child-centered nation, the United States does remarkably little for its children. Public opinion both romanticizes and demonizes children. A change in national outlook and priorities is unlikely to occur quickly. Undoubtedly the quest for ever-diminishing resources will only exacerbate the tension between generations and between advocates for social service, mental health, education, and other groups serving vulnerable populations.

The Global Epidemic

The inequitable distribution of scarce resources is a global problem, just as HIV is a global epidemic. The problems of orphans of the HIV epidemic differ in scale in other areas of the world but are part of a whole. The World Health Organization (WHO) estimates that there will be ten million AIDS orphans worldwide by the year 2000.[44] Because the HIV epidemic in Africa (as in most other areas of the world) started as and has remained a heterosexual epidemic, and because fertility is higher than in the United States, the number of children surviving AIDS in their families is extremely large. In Uganda, for example, there are already between 140,000 and 300,000 AIDS-orphaned children (up to the age of fifteen); by the year 2000 the number will be between 330,000 and 700,000. Zambia, Tanzania, Kenya, and Rwanda are also hard hit. In Asia, where the epidemic started later but where it has already taken a severe toll among young women, there are already between 20,000 and 25,000 youngsters orphaned by AIDS, and by the year 2000 there will be between 100,000 and 140,000.[45]

African countries have already had to face the devastating impacts of the epidemic on children. In Uganda alone, over three hundred organizations are providing direct services to orphans and their families. These services include medical care, housing, food, education (families must pay school fees), legal assistance, emotional support, clothing, recreation, skills training, and financial assistance.[46] The extended family, the mainstay of child care, is endangered because of extreme poverty, poor health, and increased burdens of care. A review of the impact of AIDS on the urban Ugandan family found that although there is a need for food and other material goods, AIDS disrupts family life in more profound, less tangible ways: "Family members move in and out of households depending on personal inclination, economic opportunity and family obligations. . . . AIDS truncates this normal pattern of mobility as the person becomes too weak to move[,] . . . result[ing] in adult children moving into their parents' home, young children being sent to relatives for care, or sick parents and siblings moving in with able-bodied adult family members. . . . [T]here must be ways that families can adapt to the loss of mobility that prevents normal patterns of family interaction in the dispersed kin network."[47]

The strain on developing countries will have an impact on the policies of the United States and other Western nations in terms of increasing requests for humanitarian aid, technical assistance, loan forgiveness, military assistance in times of political instability, loss of markets for U.S. goods, loss of access to raw materials, and the many other ways in which destabilized areas threaten the safety and welfare of their own citizens and other residents. Increasingly donor agencies from the United States will be asked to contribute to efforts to shore up the worldwide impact of HIV disease on children, while domestic programs also compete for public and private funding.

In addressing the global epidemic, as well as the domestic one, a strong theme predominates. Assistance to orphans and their families should not be a short-term project but a long-term commitment that supports local, sustainable initiatives. AIDS is a disease that is linked to social, cultural, and economic conditions. Children orphaned by the epidemic are the test of our future commitment to social stability, economic development, and respect for the dignity and worth of each individual.

Notes

1. Centers for Disease Control and Prevention, 1994, Update: Impact of the expanded AIDS surveillance case definition for adolescents and adults on case reporting—United States, 1993, *Morbidity and Mortality Weekly Report* 43: 160–161, 167–170.

2. National Institute of Allergy and Infectious Diseases, 1994, Clinical alert: Important information on the benefit of zidovudine for the prevention of the transmission of HIV from mother to infant, Bethesda, Md.: NIAID.

3. Levine, C., and G. Stein, 1994, *Orphans of the HIV epidemic: Unmet needs in six U.S. cities*, 2–3, New York: The Orphan Project.

4. Ibid., 11–23.

5. Wasser, S., M. Gwinn, and P. Fleming, 1993, Urban-nonurban distribution of HIV infection in childbearing women in the United States, *Journal of Acquired Immune Deficiency Syndrome* 6: 1035–1042.

6. Oxtoby, M. J., 1994, Vertically acquired HIV infection in the United States, in *Pediatric AIDS: The challenge of HIV infection in infants, children, and adolescents*, 2d ed., ed. P. A. Pizzo and C. M. Wilfert. Baltimore: Williams and Wilkins.

7. Rumley, R. L., and J. E. Esinhart, 1993, AIDS in rural North Carolina, *North Carolina Medical Journal* 54: 517–522.

8. Draimin, B. H., and C. Levine, 1994, Preliminary analysis of data for *In whose care and custody?* (a joint project of New York City's Division of AIDS Services and The Orphan Project, New York).

9. LSC and Associates, 1993, *Report on the lives of Chicago women and children living with HIV infection,* Chicago: LSC and Associates.

10. Caldwell, M. B., et al. and the Pediatric Spectrum of Disease Clinical Consortium, 1992, Biologic, foster, and adoptive parents: Care givers of children exposed perinatally to human immunodeficiency virus in the United States, *Pediatrics* 90: 603–607.

11. United States Bureau of the Census, 1991, *Current population reports: Marital status and living arrangements: March 1990,* series P-20, no. 450, Washington, D.C.: Government Printing Office.

12. Minkler, M., and K. M. Roe, 1993, *Grandmothers as caregivers: Raising children of the crack cocaine epidemic,* Newbury Park, Calif.: Sage Publications, 4.

13. Poe, L. M., 1992, *Black grandparents as parents,* Berkeley, Calif.: Lenora Madison Poe, 90–91.

14. Setal, A., 1993, A grandmother's view. In *A death in the family: Orphans of the HIV epidemic,* ed. C. Levine, New York: United Hospital Fund, 42.

15. Michaels, D., and C. Levine, 1992, Estimates of the number of motherless youth orphaned by AIDS in the United States, *Journal of the American Medical Association* 268: 3456–3461.

16. See, for example, Pinott, M., 1993, Custody and placement: The legal issues, in *A death in the family,* see note 14 above; D. Grodney, 1994, Programs for children and adolescents, in *AIDS and the new orphans: Coping with death,* ed. B. O. Dane and C. Levine, New York: Greenwood (in press), 140. For additional cases of adolescents caring for younger siblings because of parental AIDS, see F. R. Lee, 1993, With no parents, Ladeeta, 18, presses on, *New York Times,* April 6, 1993; and J. Lee, 1994, Violence "spreading like wildfire," *USA Today,* May 9, 1994. The Jessica Lee article describes the care of a ten-year-old boy who killed a classmate because of taunts that his mother has AIDS. The boy and two siblings were being raised by an eighteen-year-old brother.

17. Zayas, L., and K. Romano, Adolescents and parental death from AIDS. In *AIDS and the new orphans,* see note 16 above.

18. Barth, R., 1994, Shared foster care, *The Source* (newsletter of the AIA Resource Center, Berkeley, Calif.) 4 (1): 10–12.

19. Pinott, see note 16 above.

20. Centers for Disease Control, 1994, see note 1 above.

21. Gelber, R. D., and P. Kiselev, 1994, *Executive summary of ACTG 076,* Cambridge: Statistical and Data Analysis Center, Pediatric AIDS Clinical Trials Group, Harvard School of Public Health.

22. See Levine, C. The new orphans and grieving in the time of AIDS, in *AIDS and the new orphans,* see note 16 above; Goldstein, R., 1991, The implicated and the immune: Responses to AIDS in the arts and popular culture. In *A disease of society: Cultural and institutional responses to AIDS,* ed. D. Nelkin, D. Willis, and S. Parris, 17–42, New York: Cambridge University Press.

23. See, for example, N. Zmora, 1994, *Orphanages reconsidered: Child care institutions in progressive era Baltimore,* Philadelphia: Temple University Press.

24. Forer, L., 1988, Bring back the orphanage: An answer for today's children, *The Washington Monthly,* April.

25. Ladner, J., 1989, Bring back the orphanages, *Washington Post,* October 29, 1989.

26. Quoted in A. McCarthy, 1990, Orphans need homes: Bring back the orphanage, *Commonweal,* January 26, 1990, 39.

27. *Proceedings of the conference on the care of dependent children,* 1909, Washington: Government Printing Office. These proceedings are cited in P. C. English, 1984, Pediatrics and the unwanted child in history: Foundling homes, disease, and the origins of foster care in New York City, 1860 to 1920, *Pediatrics* 73: 700.

28. For examples of psychoanalytically oriented research see J. Bowlby, 1951, *Maternal care and mental health: A report prepared on behalf of the World Health Organization*, Geneva, Switzerland: World Health Organization, 1951, and New York: Schocken Books, 1966; Bowlby, J., 1969, *Attachment and loss*, New York: Basic Books; Provence, S., 1962, *Infants in institutions*, New York: International Universities Press; and Provence, S., 1983, *Working with disadvantaged parents and their children: Scientific and practice issues*, New Haven: Yale University Press.

29. Child Welfare League of America, 1991, *A blueprint for fostering infants, children, and youths in the 1990s*, Washington, D.C.: Child Welfare League of America, 4, 26.

30. See the profile on the AIDS Resource Foundation for Children in Levine and Stein, note 3 above, 42–44.

31. William Bennett, from a speech given to the National Urban League on July 30, 1990, quoted in E. Drucker, 1990, In Dickens' America, *The Networker*, November/December, 1990.

32. Webber, T. L., 1990, *Edwin Gould Academy: Basic concepts and organizational principles*, Chestnut, New York, 5.

33. Jones, C., 1993, Debate on race and adoptions is being reborn, *New York Times*, October 24, 1993.

34. Silverman, A. R., 1993, Outcomes of transracial adoption, in *Adoption: The Future of Children* 3 (1), ed. I. Schulman and R. Behrman, Los Altos, Calif.: The David and Lucille Packard Foundation, 104.

35. Cited in Silverman, see note 34 above, 106.

36. Kingsolver, B., 1993, *Pigs in heaven*, New York: HarperCollins.

37. Jones, 1993, see note 33 above.

38. Bartholet, E., 1993, *Family bonds: Adoption and the politics of parenting*, Boston: Houghton Mifflin.

39. Silverman, 1993, see note 34 above, 117.

40. Glynn, T. B., 1993, The role of race in adoption proceedings: A constitutional critique of the Minnesota preference statute, *Minnesota Law Review* 77: 925–952; Hardin, M., and J. Feller, 1992, Transracial adoption courts test same-race placement policies, *Youth Law News* 13 (4): 16.

41. Giordano, R., 1994, Foster family ties, *New York Newsday*, March 1, 1994.

42. Kennedy, R., 1994, Orphans of separatism: The painful politics of transracial adoption, *The American Prospect*, Spring 1994, 39–40.

43. I am grateful to the participants in The Orphan Project's March 3–5, 1994, symposium on "In whose care and custody: Orphans of the HIV epidemic in historical and global perspectives," for their comments on this theme. In particular, Deborah Dwork of Yale University explored this theme in the context of the fate of Jewish children in the Netherlands immediately after World War II.

44. United Nations Children's Fund, 1991, *Report on a meeting about AIDS and orphans in Africa, Florence 14/15, June 1991*, New York: United Nations Children's Fund, 6.

45. These estimates were developed by David Michaels, City University of New York Medical School, for a joint UNICEF-WHO publication.

46. Carol Levine, David Michaels, and Sara Back, unpublished material from survey for Global AIDS Policy Coalition, 1994.

47. McGrath, J., et al., 1993, AIDS and the urban family: Its impact in Kampala, Uganda, *AIDS Care* 5: 67, 69.

Chapter 12

Agenda for Action
THE EDITORS

This is not the end. It is not even the beginning of the end. But it is, perhaps, the end of the beginning.

Winston Churchill, November 10, 1942

Children living in families affected by HIV disease have much in common with children living in other situations of great hardship and challenge. Like children of war, they experience great privation and multiple losses. Many are children of the urban American ghetto, suffering the indignities of poverty and homelessness and raised in environments fraught with violence, abuse, and neglect. Many also grow up in a world where the chaos created by substance abuse and incarceration is part of the fabric of their daily existence. Like other children whose parents or siblings suffer from the ravages of catastrophic or fatal, chronic illnesses, children of families living with AIDS are forced to live with feelings of vulnerability, uncertainty, anger, loneliness, and stigmatization.

Children living in families affected by HIV disease are also unique. Unlike children of war, for example, juvenile survivors of the AIDS epidemic are not often supported in their grief by idealized societal portrayals of their dead parents. Unlike children in families affected by other fatal diseases, AIDS-affected children often fail to get the support provided by middle-class incomes and a safe place to live. The unique societal stigma imposed by an AIDS diagnosis forces the affected child to keep terrible secrets and to repress the natural need to talk and to share.

Were more than one hundred thousand children to be orphaned by a flood or an earthquake in this country, our nation would respond quickly, dramatically, and with the greatest empathy. The disaster confronting children affected by AIDS is no less than this, nor is their trauma less than that experienced by children who bear the burdens of war, or other family illness and death, or urban marginalization. The burdens these children bear are multiple, concurrent, and relentless.

It is not enough simply to acknowledge the existence of, or even to feel sympathy for, these thousands of children affected by HIV disease. Their many needs must be addressed. The following agenda for action, which is drawn in large part from the preceding chapters and is by no means all-inclusive, has three components: policy and practice, training, and research. Each component is essential; all must be addressed concurrently. It may become apparent in reviewing this agenda that many of the suggestions would also benefit non-HIV-affected youths who, for reasons of poverty, disenfranchisement, and lack of nurturing, are also needy. Readers with experiences in this arena will doubtless have their own ideas and priorities.

Policy and Practice

The lives of children and families affected by HIV disease can be markedly improved through both policy change and program enhancement. Our recommended changes, presented below, are aimed at reducing the stressors on HIV-affected children and their families, facilitating placements for children and adolescents, caring for professional caregivers, and giving voice to the children's needs through advocacy on their behalf.

In fulfilling these goals, several principles must guide both policy change and program enhancement. All services must be developmentally, culturally, and linguistically appropriate for the families they will serve. To satisfy these criteria, people from the communities to be served must be included in planning for program development and programs must maintain and build connections to the children's cultural roots and supports. Programs also must be staffed by persons who speak the language and understand the culture of the children and families to be served. Programs must become available and accessible for families living in nonurban as well as urban settings. Finally, programs must take into account the special needs of each individual child.

The first set of recommendations requires action by governmental policymakers, whereas the second requires action by service providers at the national, state, and/or local levels.

Necessary Actions by Governmental Policymakers

• Strengthen federal and state statutory protection for children affected by HIV and their caregivers by:

(a) defining *family* in any state or federal law pertaining to family preservation and support services from the child's perspective—that is, to include persons with whom the child is bonded—and in a way that recognizes and accommodates ethnic and cultural diversity;

(b) prohibiting, through federal (ADA, FHA, Rehabilitation Act, for example) and state discrimination law, any type of discrimination against any person because that person is thought to be HIV infected or has an association with someone who is infected;

(c) explicitly affirming that adolescents have the capacity to consent to (or refuse consent for) all health care and school-based health education programs, and that providers must maintain confidentiality with regard to that care;

(d) modifying existing confidentiality protection to allow limited nonconsensual disclosure of parental HIV status if such disclosure is essential to providing needed health and mental health services to that parent's child or children;

(e) recognizing (including for the purposes of financial and clinical support) a range of custody arrangements, including kinship foster care, standby guardianship, shared foster family care, and adolescent co-guardianship;

(f) ensuring equitable and adequate payments and subsidies for substitute caregivers of HIV-affected children that are comparable across classes of guardianship (foster parents, legal guardians, adoptive parents) and that provide the same support to low-income kin caregivers as is provided to non-kin caregivers;

(g) guaranteeing, at a rate of compensation sufficient to attract competent, trained counsel, legal representation for each affected child throughout the permanency planning and custody transfer process and expediting all judicial proceedings involving that child's care and custody;

(h) restoring the private right of action to enforce states' compliance with the AACWA's "reasonable efforts" requirement.

• Condition receipt of applicable existing and new federal funds on (or provide federal financial incentives for):

(a) the adoption of state laws that provide the statutory protection outlined above;

(b) states' development and implementation of comprehensive health education programs;

(c) state- and community-based mechanisms to ensure that affected children and their families receive coordinated, efficient care from AIDS service organizations and medical, child welfare, education, and mental health providers.

• Relax regulations that strictly limit the number of children placed with one foster or adoptive family so that siblings from a family affected by HIV can be placed together when appropriate. For children who be must placed temporarily in foster care because of a parent's HIV-related hospitalization, facilitate placements in the child's home community and relax restrictions on the duration of such voluntary placements.

• Better enforce existing protection against HIV-related discrimination through:

    (a) more aggressive monitoring by government civil rights agencies;

    (b) prompt resolution of disputes in a manner that protects litigants' privacy;

    (c) full relief to those who prove discrimination, including compensatory and punitive damages and attorneys' fees.

• Enhance the services available to affected children and their caregivers by:

    (a) extending eligibility for and ensuring access to family preservation and support services for the HIV-affected child's second family (kinship, foster, adoptive), as well as the child's original family;

    (b) extending Medicaid eligibility—until the enactment of universal health care coverage—to all HIV-affected children in families living at or below 250 percent of federal poverty level and increasing the number of full-service school-based health clinics;

    (c) vigorously enforcing Medicaid mandates, such as EPSDT.

• Ensure adequate funding for:

    (a) sufficient personnel to ensure expeditious custody transfers (legal services attorneys for low income families, child welfare staff to do home studies, and probate court judges, for example);

    (b) discretionary financial aid to meet the low-income new guardian's immediate needs in assuming care (to purchase an additional bed, for example);

    (c) supportive services for affected children and all new low-income caregivers (respite care, family support services, family preservation services, and mental health services, for example);

    (d) financial subsidies (for renting a larger apartment, for example) for low-income guardians who are not part of the foster care or preadoptive systems;

(e) organizing and conducting regional and national conferences targeted to this population;

(f) newsletters and other publications designed to encourage families and providers to build and join natural support groups.

• Eliminate restrictions on information sharing and the pooling of funds when an affected child and his or her family are eligible for benefits from more than one agency.

• Ensure that the National AIDS Clearinghouse and other federally supported national databases include (and make easily available to all caregivers) information on programs working on behalf of affected children and youths.

• Establish as a federal funding priority empirical research on the psychosocial impacts of HIV disease on HIV-affected children. Insist that federal funding for such research be used effectively by building on existing psychosocial research on at-risk children to the extent possible and by encouraging collaborative research efforts.

Necessary Actions by Service Providers at the National, State, and Local Levels

Clinical and Support Programs for Children and Families

• Develop identification, assessment, and referral programs for affected children and youths who are at risk of or who are experiencing mental health problems in response to parental HIV-related illness.

• Establish developmentally and culturally appropriate programs for children and youths to:

(a) help them to cope with a parent's chronic illness;

(b) help them and their families decide what and when to tell others;

(c) foster parent-child communication.

• Establish early permanency planning programs that:

(a) help the infected parents in their decision to initiate planning;

(b) include in decisions regarding care and custody those members of a child's extended family with whom the child feels a sense of attachment;

(c) help identify a second "family";

(d) assist both the original and second families with custody, placement, and mental health issues (such as loss, bereavement, helping ill parents to relinquish parental responsibility to another family);

(e) refer the original family to legal services to initiate the transfer in custody;

(f) advise potential second families (kin and non-kin) about differences between the status of private guardianship and that of licensed foster care or adoption regarding state involvement and access to entitlements;

(g) link the child and his or her second family to follow-up services (financial, health, mental health, for example).

• Create supportive environments for bereavement and healing for children, their families, and their caretakers, using a range of therapeutic models and tools (for example, peer support groups, school- and community-based bereavement groups, telephone support groups, individual, family, and group counseling services, summer camps, and personal life history books and videotapes to maintain links to the child's past).

• Develop specialized mentoring programs for HIV-affected children and youths to provide:

(a) ongoing, consistent, nurturing individual attention throughout parental illness and after the parent's death;

(b) help in decision making;

(c) advocacy on their behalf with schools, social service and health providers, and state authorities.

• Ensure that clinicians working with HIV-affected families have access to competent clinical consultation and supervision to help them to:

(a) better understand the initial reticence of families to engage in services;

(b) cope with the impact of working with a caseload of patients, all of whom are actively involved with death and dying;

(c) better bear the child's negative emotions, including rage at abandonment;

(d) manage the boundaries of clinical interviews in crowded home settings.

Health Services for Affected Children

• Develop and implement comprehensive, skills-based, accurate, and developmentally and culturally appropriate health education (teen pregnancy, STD, substance abuse education) programs in schools, at sites that provide residential care to youths, and in community-based agencies serving out-of-school youths. Develop school curricula that acknowledge the impact of this epidemic on students' lives.

• Increase the number of school-based health clinics offering a full range of health services.

Placements

• Develop voluntary, transitional placements for children and youths in their own communities while a parent is episodically hospitalized to afford continuity in the child's schooling and social supports.

• Develop and support family-based placement resources that maintain, as therapeutically appropriate, the sibling unit and positive connections to the child's friends, schools, and natural community supports.

• Establish financial support mechanisms for new caregivers that are equitable and adequate.

Specialized Services for Adolescents

• Develop workplace training, mentoring programs, and sports and arts programs for adolescents who survive AIDS in their families to assist them in their transition to adulthood.

• Provide adolescent guardians with skill-building training in parenting and in family communication, and with ongoing professional backup support to assist them in responding to the developmental and psychosocial needs of their siblings.

• Assist youths with family caretaking responsibilities to locate alternative educational programs that are sensitive to their unique needs (a flexible school schedule, for example).

• Enhance the variety and adequacy of placement options for adolescents who have no available family placement resource by developing:

   (a) specialized therapeutic foster care placements;

   (b) specialized therapeutic residential programs;

   (c) supported transitional housing opportunities;

   (d) supervised independent living programs.

Case Management

• Develop case management services that include legal, social work/mental health, and entitlement specialists. Provide case management services to both original and second families, as needed.

• For children and families who need services from several agencies, establish a single case manager who links the family with all formal service providers. Co-locate needed services within a "one-stop" model of care to the extent possible.

Care for Formal Caregivers

• Develop and implement programs that provide clinicians and other formal caregivers who serve affected children with peer support and clinical consultation and supervision. Provide for rotation in caregivers' assignments.

Training

A whole generation of professionals in a multiplicity of disciplines needs to be trained and in some instances retrained to understand and develop sensitivities for the complex array of challenges unique to this population of children. Parents, relatives, and other caregivers also can benefit from an enhanced understanding of the needs of these children. Among the programs that must be initiated are:

• Training for parents (in individual and group settings) and for medical caregivers to help them to come to terms with what these affected children already know and to help them give the children the language with which to talk about it.

• Training for parents and other caregivers, and for attorneys, social workers, and judges who are assisting families in making permanent custody arrangements, about the course of HIV disease, children's reactions to illness and death, government entitlements, and custody options to:

   (a) enhance understanding of the importance of timing and pacing in the custody planning process and of involving family, broadly defined, in the process;

   (b) assure the children placements that best meet their short- and long-term needs.

• Training for teachers, social workers, attorneys, juvenile justice and family court personnel, and other professionals likely to work with these children, about HIV disease and its impact on the uninfected child to:

   (a) identify special needs and behavioral symptoms of family crisis and foster an awareness that disturbing behaviors may be a reaction to these stresses;

   (b) assure proper evaluations;

(c) promote appropriate referrals to community services, especially mental health services;

(d) influence the type of treatment offered (for example, to encourage intensive follow-up, job skills training, and bereavement counseling when these youths are released into the community from juvenile justice facilities).

• Training for clinicians regarding the importance of initiating a care plan, making tangible efforts to accept and support the patient, and offering a generous commitment to treatment without the expectation of an immediate reciprocal response from the patient or clear evidence that the patient/family will take immediate responsibility for his or her care (an approach different from the more familiar mental health evaluation and treatment experience).

• Training for all professionals who work with these children and/or their families concerning:

(a) the importance of working with the multigenerational family system of both the birth and chosen family so they can function as a resource for the affected child;

(b) the principles of resilience, so external environments can be structured in ways that maximize the likelihood of positive child development and successful coping;

(c) the contribution of cultural and religious beliefs to family decisions and functioning, so the professionals will develop and demonstrate respect for this diversity;

(d) the importance of providing natural support and mental health resources to families and their children before problems (including who will care for children after death of the parent) reach crisis levels;

(e) the need for information sharing and reductions in redundant services (multiple case managers, for example) so families are not additionally burdened and resources are used most efficiently.

• Training and peer support groups for clinicians working in HIV/AIDS mental health programs concerning issues of death and dying and managing personal feelings of frustration and hopelessness.

Research

Qualitative as well as quantitative research about the impact of AIDS on the uninfected children is crucial. Well-controlled longitudinal studies, in particular, can allow us to more accurately measure their experience against that of children who suffer other parental and sibling deaths and better assess which components of the children's responses are AIDS-specific. Such research must confront formidable methodologic challenges, including small sample sizes, a paucity of basic research concerning how the family is structured and how it functions within and across those communities most affected by AIDS, reliance on instruments of unproven validity and reliability for the minority and ethnic populations that must be studied, and the need to provide incentives to reduce loss to follow-up and maximize data.[1] We clearly cannot postpone responding to the needs of these children, however, while we await the results of such well-controlled, methodologically pure studies. Research must occur concurrently. New discoveries should continuously inform and guide changes in policy and practice. Five general areas for research have been proposed by the authors in this volume. Each encompasses a range of research questions, which include:

Numbers of Children Affected

• How many children in the United States and worldwide have already lost or will lose mothers, fathers, siblings, and other loved ones to AIDS? Over what period of time?

• How many children, and of what ages, will need placements through our foster care system in the short term? In the long term?

Telling the Children

• How, when, and what are children told about HIV in their families, and what role does culture play in this decision?

• What is the extent of children's understanding of HIV in their families, even when they have not been told?

• How do children react to being told, and what factors modify this reaction, positively and negatively?

Children's Experience Living with AIDS in the Family

• What is the impact of AIDS in the family on the day-to-day life of the uninfected children—attending school, accompanying visits to medical providers, remaining home to care for younger siblings, and so on?

• How do uninfected children react in the short and long term to parental and sibling illnesses and deaths from AIDS? How do these reactions differ if the child experiences multiple AIDS-related losses? How do such factors as the child's age, culture, socioeconomic status, and family relationships modify these reactions? To what extent are these reactions specific to and attributable to the dynamics of living within a family coping with the stigmatizing and debilitating illness of AIDS, rather than to the other stresses common to many families now living with AIDS?

• How do children's reactions differ, if at all, if the illness has been *named* as AIDS? If it has not been *named*? What implications do these findings have for clinical support of parents?

• What proportion of uninfected adolescents become teenage parents at about the time of AIDS-related deaths in their families? What are the motivations for such early pregnancies and what are the implications for AIDS and teen pregnancy–prevention efforts?

• What are the possible protective factors that might be operating for children who appear to be symptomless in response to these AIDS-related losses?

Placement and Custody

• Who most commonly cares for the child during the parents' illnesses and hospitalizations? After the parents' deaths? How do these caretaking arrangements differ in families in which there is a child who is also infected by HIV?

• In how many and what types of families do teenagers and young adults assume care of younger brothers and sisters? What are the long-term effects of this caretaking for the adolescent "parent"? For the younger siblings? What supportive services are most helpful to these older adolescents?

• What factors influence the timing of custody planning? How can we best encourage parents of every cultural background to make timely custody plans?

• How often do siblings remain together after parental deaths? For how long? What factors contribute to sibling separations?

• What roles do culture, religious beliefs, socioeconomic status, and current entitlement, guardianship, foster care, and adoption laws and agency practice play in influencing placement choices?

• How stable are the placements over an extended period of time, and what influences their stability? What are the positive coping strategies second families successfully employ? What supportive interventions best promote good outcomes, continuity, and family and/or sibling cohesiveness in the children's new placements?

• What supportive services are most helpful to grandmothers who assume care of grandchildren while mourning the deaths of their own children and, possibly, other grandchildren?

• What are the consequences of long-term co-parenting (which occurs when the sole remaining parent, who has chosen a new guardian for her child, lives longer than expected) on these adolescent survivors and their younger siblings?

• What is the appropriate role, if any, of residential care as a placement option? What services must be provided to make it a placement which furthers the best interests of children?

Interventions to Help Children

• What are the optimum therapeutic approaches to take with these children to help them understand and cope with their feelings? How might these approaches be unique to AIDS (differing, that is, from those used with children whose lives are affected by losses associated with other parental illnesses, neglect, parental substance abuse)?

• What home-based or community interventions are most effective in enabling these children to regain, or continue to encounter, supportive childhood experiences that foster their resilience?

• What are the short- and long-term effects of some of the therapeutic interventions currently being used (child and adolescent bereavement, support groups and individual counseling, for example)?

• How well informed are AIDS-affected adolescents about the linkages between unsafe sexual behavior, drug use behavior, and AIDS? How can we improve our risk reduction education for this specific group of adolescents, who may be engaging in risky behavior in part as a reaction to familial losses?

• Can adolescents who have successfully survived transition into new families serve as mentors to other adolescents during their transition?

• What appear to be the positive coping strategies that help families manage the stresses of AIDS-related illnesses? How best can we foster and build on these?

• How do we most effectively and efficiently develop and provide services within nonurban areas? In underserved communities?

• How can we enhance public understanding and support for this population of children and assure secure funding (rather than just demonstration grants) for services to meet their needs?

• What are the likely consequences of our failing to meet the needs of these children and youths? Absent intervention, what proportion of these youths will engage in behaviors that will prove costly to them and to society (delinquent behavior, teen pregnancy)?

When Winston Churchill observed, more than a half-century ago, "it is perhaps the end of the beginning," he was speaking of the great conflagration—World War II—that then engulfed the world. As with the worldwide pandemic of AIDS, there seemed to be no end in sight. We now know, however, that when Churchill made these remarks, the end of the war was less than three years away. Would that the end of AIDS were so close. Because it is not, our challenge is to work together to decrease the spread of HIV disease and to care for all of those whose lives it touches.

Note

1. These and other methodologic challenges are discussed more fully in the June, 1994 Supplement of the *Journal of Developmental and Behavioral Pediatrics,* ed. L. Bauman and L. Wiener. This Supplement also identifies gaps in current research concerning children and families affected by HIV disease.

Part Four

Voices:
Children, Parents, and
Caregivers

The Reverberating Themes

The previous chapters have discussed, from a scholarly vantage point, the many challenges that confront children living with HIV disease in their families, but the children's own voices, joined with those of their parents and other caregivers, argue far more poignantly. These voices passionately echo many of this book's themes. Together with the words and pictures that made up the first part of this book, the following selections—written by children, parents, a grandmother, and a foster/adoptive mother—form a full chorus of voices of families affected by HIV disease.

As noted in the Introduction, three themes weave through this chorus and through the thoughts expressed in the preceding chapters: the challenges that HIV disease presents to the uninfected child; the uninfected child's response to these challenges; and society's response to these children.

Challenges to the Children

Among the challenges that HIV disease presents to the uninfected child, the most prominent are the uncertainty and the profound changes and losses that HIV brings to their lives and the silence that societal stigma forces them to keep.

As discussed in Chapters 2 and 4, uncertainty is an essential feature of the lives of children living with HIV disease in their families. Because AIDS is a chronic but fatal disease accompanied by unpredictable episodes of acute illness, parents struggling with their own disease and/or with disease in their partners and children have great difficulty providing their uninfected children the "secure base" they need to develop into competent adults. Significant changes in the home lives of these children, and eventually even in their custody, are inevitable. For each child born into the family, there is uncertainty whether the baby is infected or not. The artwork of these children, presented earlier in this volume, depicts this uncertainty and unpredictability through human figures who float unanchored, adrift, and in limbo. The unexpectedness of her mother's death was something with which Onivea continued to struggle a year later (see her March 22 and April 19 journal entries). Uncertainty is also a central theme of "My Life," a brief essay by a fifteen-year-old boy orphaned by AIDS.

Multiple losses also pose extraordinary challenges to these children. As Chapter 7 emphasizes, the losses suffered by these children are comparable in magnitude to those suffered by children in war: losses of parents, of siblings, of homes. The children's work, especially Onivea's journal and JR's picture, captures the impact of these losses. Three of the narratives that follow provide an adult perspective. Matthew eloquently describes the inevitable path of loss that all those with HIV disease must travel. Ann's narrative, too, speaks of her fears not only of losing her health and life, but of being required to sell the family home to pay for health care. The narrative by Grace eloquently suggests that losses may not end for these children even after they have been orphaned and moved into adoptive homes.

Society's stigmatizing response to HIV disease also presents great challenges to the uninfected child, as noted in Chapters 4 and 9. Fears of ostracism and loss of family support figure prominently in the writing by Kara in Part One, as well as in the writings that follow by Ann, Matthew, Grace, and Marva. As we saw in Chapter 2, infected adults often respond either by not telling their children about the disease, lying to them about its cause, or telling them and then requiring that they also keep the secret. These themes of secrecy and of the child's resulting feelings of isolation and loneliness, discussed in Chapters 4, 5, and 7, are echoed in the writings by Ann and Matthew that follow.

The Child's Response

The child's response to the uncertainty, losses, stigma, secrecy, and isolation that HIV disease brings is varied. Some children are resilient, for the reasons discussed in Chapters 7 and 10. "My Life" is a self-portrait of one such resilient child, who, despite being orphaned by AIDS, is a straight-A student at age fifteen. Other children, like the young girl who writes "I Miss You," experience problems in school. Some youngsters may try to protect their parents. The young girl whose narrative starts "My life has not been very easy" admitted to a crime she did not commit to spare her infected father a prison term. Other, older children will often assume parental roles, as discussed by many of the authors, and as poignantly illustrated in two of this volume's earlier drawings, "Me on the Outside, Me on the Inside" and "I'm Real Good Because My Mamma is Sick and Might Die." Two of the narratives that follow provide contrasting views of this response: Marva heartily supports her granddaughter's role as the new "mother" of her nuclear family, whereas Ann criticizes those who urged her young son to become the "man of the house" when her husband died. As described in Chapters 3 and 7 and as illustrated in Onivea's March 30 journal entry, children may also feel responsible for the illness that has befallen the family. Their feelings of guilt mirror those of their parents. As Matthew stresses in his narrative, "The guilt is incredible. . . ."

Our Response to the Children

The needs of children who survive AIDS in their families are formidable. To date, our response to these needs has been meager. Many of these children need a new home, often with family, sometimes with strangers. As noted by nearly all of this volume's authors, identifying appropriate new families and planning for placement are difficult tasks that are only made harder by existing law and by current policy and practice of child welfare agencies. The vignettes that follow illustrate the range of response to placement dilemmas. Ann, like Kara, writes of having no good option for her children. Marva's account illustrates the important role that grandmothers often play in these families, and the burdens that this role imposes on them. Grace's journal gives a glimpse of the possibilities for creative, and planned, transitions in guardianship that place the needs of children ahead of the needs of their adult caretakers. Grace writes as well about some of the pressures felt by those involved in transracial placements, discussed in Chapters 6 and 11. Grace and Marva's chronicles give personal voice to the need to "care for the caretakers," an issue addressed in Chapters 7 and 11. Marva's story, in particular, illustrates the skip-generation parenting described in Chapter 11: following the death of her daughter-in-law to AIDS, "mothering" responsibility for the eight children in the family was assumed by Marva and by the eighteen-year-old eldest daughter in the family. Marva's account also illustrates the important role family elders can play in providing links to the past for these children, a role described in Chapter 7 as essential for healing. Finally, the narratives by Ann, Matthew, and Grace illustrate a few of the failures in the response of our existing social services systems to these children and their families. As can be seen in every chapter, AIDS presents enormous and as yet unmet challenges to the child welfare, mental health, education, and legal systems and to our faith communities. The voices of these children, parents, and caregivers call out to us to begin to meet these challenges.

The Voices of Children

The following three selections were written by youths who were between twelve and fifteen years old. The following brief descriptions provide some contextual information about the young authors.

I Miss You

"I Miss You" is a poem written by a twelve-year-old girl. Her father has AIDS and is in and out of her life. A trusted adult went to her principal and teacher to explain her behavior. When the adult told them vaguely that the girl's father was very sick and "dying of a disease that is now prevalent in the community," the principal replied, "Don't tell me that I have a child in the school with AIDS because all my teachers will quit." Her teacher commented that the "problem" was this child's to bear alone. When a fellow student experienced the death of a family member by a shooting, however, the death was discussed in class, and there was appropriate grief and response from the teacher and classmates. Frustrated that school is not available to her as a support, the girl literally screams at her teacher in her rage. The poem reflects this rage, as well as her anticipatory grief for her father's death.

I MISS YOU

I Miss you so my body
cries out.
In my heart I scream
AND PouT.
I say AND pray. I miss
you So
But then I said you
had to go.
As my heart sinks to
the ground. I Lie in my
room I weep And frown.
I try to Keep you in the past
But in my Heart you'll ALways LAst.

My Life Has Not Been Very Easy

The fourteen-year-old girl who wrote this is extremely attached to her father, who has AIDS. Her mother is not infected but gets hysterical and does not protect her from her father's abuse. Her father even sold her precious bicycle to buy drugs although when he was well he used to go bike riding with her often. She feels very protective of him and feels his potential loss very intensely. This girl was recently arrested. Her father had hidden his drugs in her dresser drawer, and when the police raided their home and asked her if it was her dresser and her drugs, she said "Yes." She later explained that she assumed the guilt to protect her father because she didn't want him to die in jail.

My life has not been very easy but I Deal with it. I want you to Know that you Don4 have to feel Sorry for me but I expect you to under stand where I'm coming from and where I am going. I'v had to deal with seeing my dad in the hospital sick thinking will he die but I also seen him having fun riding bike with me and helping me with my home work. I just hope to see him in the future and be helping my kids with their homework and ride bike. Maybe soon in the future they will come up with a cure for this Disease.

My Life

This essay was written by a fifteen-year-old boy. Both of his parents have died of AIDS. Though his mother actively used drugs, she was very loving and encouraged him to excel, and doing well in school is a positive feature in his life. He and a sister maintained straight-A averages the whole time their mother was using drugs and while she was sick and dying, and they continue to do so. He dreams of becoming a doctor and was recently accepted into a college-track premed program in his high school. The oldest child in the family, this youth cares for his two younger siblings in the home of an aunt who has four children of her own. He is desperately seeking a job to help support the new family. His aunt, who feels overburdened, cannot be a maternal figure to him, a situation that exacerbates his feelings of loss for his mother. Note, in particular, how the boy signed his essay.

My life

My life hes been good
For the First 10 years I had a
Loving mother and my Family lived very
close to each other. My mother was a
very good mather and I new that
she loved us very much. When I
turned 11 on June 9th 1999 I had
a wonderfull birthday but like a
week later My mother got really sick. I
did not now what was going on I was
scared because the ambulance came
and my brother and sister were
crying. I was not crying because I
was so to scared and did'nt now
what was going on. When my mother
came out the hospital she look
very tired and sick so I asked her
what was wrong and she said
mommy got sick so I Left it at that,
but my mom seem like she was
getting sick like every other week
and I did't now what
was wrong but I now my mother

was sick. So like the third month
when we move from the terrace
to willem street my mom seem week
and could not really get around.
then a couple of month
passed and my birthday came up and
I turned 12. I asked her on my
birthday what was wrong and she
said I think your old enough and I'm
going to tell you what was wrong
she said that she was effected
with AIDS and I said what was that
she said it's a virus and that it is
a very dangerous virus and she may die
in a few months. I was stuned
because I could not beleive that my
mother was going to die the only
person that nurised me when I was
sick and she told me and my brothers
and sisters that if we wanted to
make her happy was to stay in
school and get an education and she will
be the happiest mother in the world.
I started crying and she hugged me
and said that every thing would be

all right becouse aunty ~~there~~ would
be there for us and that she
will not let anything happen to
us and that if anything do happen
to her she would still be with us
in our heart. I said all right and I
will try to be strong for my ~~brother~~
and sisters. 7 to 8 months later my mother
died of AIds she lived to be 28 years
old. Now I am 14 going on 15 and ~~as~~ me my
brother and sister is living with our aunt
and every thing is all right for us.
~~and~~ My aunt treat us like we were
hers and I love her very much

by: S.O.S
o n p
m e e
e C
i
a
l

The Voices of Parents and Caregivers

"Matthew"

Matthew is in his mid-thirties and the father of a five-year-old son. Until recently, he was the director of two residences for persons with AIDS. In the eight months that have elapsed since he told his story, he has been episodically quite ill.

Whether you're an individual with HIV disease or you're a family where the child or the primary caregiver, mother, father has AIDS, the losses that come about are just so devastating and are not being taken care of. . . . What's missing is some centralized effort, governmental or otherwise, some resources that can take care of those losses for people. I can address that as a professional who runs programs for people with AIDS, mostly housing programs with services wrapped around the people, or as an individual with HIV disease who has a five-year-old son. I often think about it on both of those levels.

If I was to get sick tomorrow, just as any of my clients who have full-blown AIDS, one by one I lose things. I lose my job, because I can't do it anymore. I lose my income because I'm not working. I lose my insurance. I lose my home and my son loses his home with me. . . . He starts to lose the support of me, as his father. I start becoming too weak to give him the things he needs from a father, and little by little I end up with nothing. So, at the end of this chain of events, you have Matthew with basically nothing. You have his five year old son witnessing this whole, awful, terrible dilemma and being traumatized by it. Christopher, that's my son's name. Where does he go? If I die, where does he go? Who takes care of him? Who is his father? While I'm sick and dying, where do I live? Do I have a family that will fill in those gaps? If I don't [have a family], the system that exists is totally inadequate. People should not live in a shelter, whether it's a family shelter or an individual shelter. That's not dignified. You don't get the appropriate health care, you don't get the appropriate nutrition. It's not the kind of place you should live if you're healthy, so if you have AIDS it's certainly not a place to live.

The bottom line is really the tremendous losses that people suffer because of AIDS, and the losses that the children suffer are so much more deep and magnified. . . . People think it happens in Africa, it happens in Haiti, it happens, you know, in underdeveloped countries, but it doesn't happen in the United States. Well, it happens here on a major scale. . . .

Sometimes I look at my son and, you know, it just grieves me terribly to think that I won't be there later on in life, to be his father, to take care of him and to teach him the things that he needs to learn. He doesn't know what AIDS is; he doesn't understand HIV. And I have not discussed it with him at this point. I think that if I was sick, I would be talking to him about being ill, and talking about the future. But for right now, while I'm well and healthy, I don't need to discuss it with him. As he gets older, I certainly intend to educate him about HIV and people with AIDS.

He's spent time with me at the [AIDS] residence, and his reaction is really amazing. He witnessed one of our residents, who was dying, and he witnessed an ambulance come and take this guy to the hospital. At the time, I think he was three and a half or four years. He had never seen the guy before. The guy's name was Bill. And he just sat there and stared and watched as the ambulance came, and they couldn't resuscitate Bill, so they had to put him in a blanket and lift him out. And it was a really horrendous scene, and Bill was skin and bones. . . . He was vomiting. . . . And my son watched them bring him out, and he turned to me and said, "What's the matter with Bill?" And I said, "He's very sick." And he said, "Is he going to come back?" And I said, "I don't think so." And he said, "Is he going to die?" This is a three-and-a-half- to four-year-old kid. And I said, "He probably will die." And that was it. He never said another word that whole day. This is going on two years now since Bill died. And every time he comes to the house, he asks me, "When's Bill coming back? When's Bill coming back?" And I tell him, "He's not coming back. He died." And yet he always asks me, "When's Bill coming back? When's Bill coming back?" And it's really strange that a three-and-a-half-year-old would just see a guy once, and those are the things that stick out in their minds. If it was to happen to his father, I just, you know, it kills me to think what's going to stick out in his mind.

The guilt is incredible. . . . I feel guilty because I became infected and therefore I might die and leave my son without a father. I feel guilty because I became infected and it has to affect my child's life. No matter how I play it, he's going to be affected by my positivity. Even if I don't end up with AIDS, he's still going to be affected. If somebody [reads] that I'm HIV and they figure out who I am and my son's relationship, it will affect him. . . . If I'm dying and my son had to witness that . . . just like some of the residents [where I work] are dying and their children have to witness that . . . it's a mess. It's a disaster. It's pain and suffering and it's loss; and there are no agencies that step in and make it better. No money that steps in and makes it easier. There's people like myself and other professionals . . . that are in the field, but we're a drop in the bucket.

If I was talking to Christopher now, I would just tell him how much I love him. And I would tell him about AIDS. I would try to tell Christopher to not make the same mistakes that I made in my life, and try to teach him about the important things in life. . . . Such as loving, loving and not hating, not judging people but taking care of people and giving.

Marva

Marva is a woman in her late fifties, living with her husband, who has two sons with HIV disease, a daughter-in-law who has died of AIDS, and eight grandchildren for whom she is now a primary source of support.

Somebody's gotta start educating people about HIV, because these are human beings we're talking about—like sons and daughters and nieces and nephews . . . and we need to let them know that they are loved. They are God's creatures . . . not an outcast to society—and that's the way that they make you feel, as if you were an outcast, you know. . . . These are my children that they're talking about.

When I lost my daughter-in-law [Olive], that was the hardest, 'cause the little children were there. It was eight little kids. So it was a lot of responsibility on me. . . . They didn't understand what was happening to their mother. They didn't take her death very easily in the beginning. They got counseling, and they're doing a lot better now in school. Their grades are good. They're beautiful children. And thank God they're free of the virus.

I also found out that God will bring you through. He will walk you right through it. All you gotta do is just trust him. He just like take you by the hand and pull you right through it. And I didn't do that when my son first got sick. I was trying to handle it all by myself. The visiting nurses would come and I was so proud. I wouldn't even let them help me change him or bathe him. "I'll do it. I'll bathe him. I'll take care of him." They said, "Don't do that, that's my job." I said, "Well, yeah, but that's my son."

One Sunday, after coming home from church, my older son told me, "You had a telephone call, Mommy." I said, "Who was it?" He says, "Tony called." And I said, "OK, he'll probably call me back." He called back, and he told me, "Mommy, Olive have AIDS, full blown AIDS, and I'm HIV-positive." And I felt like a hole had opened up and swallowed me. . . . I just couldn't believe it. . . . Until I went down there the next day. And I took one look at her, and I said, "You coming home with me." And a couple of weeks later, they moved up here with me. I had all eight of them. My husband, my daughters, all of us, we was in one house. But I got her help. I started taking her to the doctors. I did every-thing I could for her. Because her family rejected her—they just plain out rejected her and I just couldn't do it because she was my daughter-in-law.

You know, we have an old saying that God doesn't put on us

anymore than we can bear. You learn that you can *take a lot* if you have to—you can *do* a lot if you have to—that you don't just have to fold up—and give up—if you can just find the strength to keep going. And eventually things get a little bit better, and you know it's not the end of the world. I got beautiful grandchildren. I hope Tony lives to see them grown. I hope God lets me live long enough to see them grown. There's eight beautiful children there. And five of them are my step[grand]children, but they're so close to me it's just like they're my own children—my own children you know. And they love me, and I love them. So . . . that's the part that keeps me going—for them—I have to keep going for my grandchildren.

I tell them that if anything should happen to their dad, that I'm there. And I tell them I will never let anybody separate them. And I tell them that if I have to we will all live in that three-bedroom house together. I don't want them to have to ever feel like they're gonna have to be separated. Because they're very close children. See, they're very, very close kids. They're not, like, they don't *like* one another, they *love* one another. . . . Peggy is eighteen years old, and I always tell them—I get very indignant with them when they don't mind her, because she *is* the mamma. I'm just the grandma. *She's* the mamma. Because she does everything that a mother would do. She's just that concerned about them. It's a lot of responsibility for an eighteen-year-old. So I say to her sometimes, you want to come and stay the weekend with me—just so she can get away from them for a little while?

I never went to counseling. I had another way of getting counseling. My husband takes me fishing every Saturday. I found out it was cheaper to talk to the fish than it was to talk to doctors, 'cause the fish don't charge me nothing. So we would go fishing every Saturday, all day, and pack a lunch. . . . I never thought AIDS or HIV that whole time I was out there fishing. But when I got back home, it would start all over again. It was rough. It still is rough.

One day . . . I'll call her Miss Ruby, 'cause she's named after my Mamma so I figure with a name like that you should show a little respect, and Miss Ruby she came to me and she said they wanted to know where their daddy was. And I told them where he was. And she looked and she says, "Oh, if Daddy go up to God where Mommy is, then we won't have no Mommy and we won't have no Daddy." And that really got to me. That was the tear-jerker for me. Because I didn't expect a little five-year-old to say that to me. And she'll talk about her mother, and she'll hear a song and she'll sing that song. She's the baby, but she talks about her more than the other ones. But I don't let any of them forget her. I say, "Boy, she sure would have liked this." I try to keep her memory fresh in their minds, because I talk to them about their mother all the time. I don't want them to ever forget her. . . . We look at pictures together. We look at pictures and point out each thing and what she was doing. And I try to do those things with those little kids. Because they don't have anybody but me to do that with. When it comes to being grandmother, I'm like the grandmother and the momma. And I'm not as young as I used to be, and it takes a little more out of me, but I have to do it. . . . One day, they're gonna be grown. . . . And that's my daily prayer, just let us live long enough so that they can take care of themselves and won't nobody have to take care of them.

There's life after HIV. I thought it was the end of the world, but it's not. Life goes on. I didn't think that way for a long time. . . . I'd come home in the morning, and I think I must have begged God all day long, "Please don't take my child." That was everyday. Go to sleep on my knees, praying "God please don't take my baby. Please let him live." And one day, I compromised with him. I made bargains with him. "If you don't take him, if you let him live, I'll do this. . . ." And one day after, I realized that, some people lost their babies when they were first born. Some of them never even got a chance to have 'em alive. I said, "I've had him for thirty-three years." And I said, "you have a lot to be thankful for." So I changed my prayer, and I said, "God, I'm not gonna ask you that anymore. That was wrong." And I said, "I have a new prayer. Everyday that you let me have him, I'll be thankful. If it's one day, two days, whatever." Everyday, because this is the day that the Lord has made, and whatever day it is, I'll be grateful. If he decides that, OK, it's no more for Tony, then I can live with that. Because he's forty years old now. He's not thirty-three. I thanked him for everyday that he let me have him. So that's the way that I get through things.

HIV and AIDS, it's our disease. It's not just my disease, it's everybody in here disease. It's not just a gay person's disease, an HIV-person's disease. It's our disease. It's everybody's disease. I know there's gonna be many, many more [people with family members who are sick] and everybody's story will be a little different from mine. . . . But they're true stories. . . . It's the truth. It's the truth. And the truth will set you free.

"Grace"

Grace is a mother, a grandmother, and now also a foster and adoptive mother. She lives in a large, old house with thirteen children, all of whose lives have been changed by AIDS. She shares parts of her journal, and the story of one of her children.

When people ask me what got me into doing foster care I think they expect me to give an answer that will make them exclaim, "Oh, but of course!" Actually, my reasons are much more vague. In part, it's because I've always wanted a large family. And I have enough material things in life to share. And there's room in my heart for more kids.

When I was a kid there were orphanages. I visited one once, and remember kids with vacant eyes and pajamas on at 2 p.m. Later, as an adult, I remember boarder babies in hospitals with only TV sets for company. My folks grew up in the Depression. They said kids without homes were not their problem. But I believe I am my brother's keeper.

Agencies sometimes advertise their need for foster families. Why did I actually respond to the ad and call the agency? I think in part it's because I discussed the whole idea with my son, and like any seven year old, he didn't let me forget it. I was afraid. But he didn't know that, and he did know a good idea, like children often do.

Dealing with a fatal illness, especially one carrying the stigma that AIDS does, isn't easy, but I have not ever regretted it. You learn how to keep secrets, never even discussing diagnosis with close friends for fear of losing them. You gradually find your circle of friends is smaller because you've eliminated the people who unwittingly have shown their prejudice toward people with AIDS.

•   •   •

March, 1991

I'm still getting mostly nowhere in trying to adopt Kenny. His lawyer and social worker seem to accomplish nothing, and I wonder if they even try. I think they want to save their time and effort because they don't understand how important it is to die as an adopted child rather than a ward of the state. They try to humor me by saying they will do a living will with his birth mother. Then the lawyer says that of course a living will has no real power. As if I already didn't know that.

So two weeks ago I ordered [all the kids] engraved pencils, mostly to eliminate the fighting over who owns which pencil. I ordered the one for Kenny engraved as Kenny Jones Somma. When the pencils arrived he was tickled to see his last name changed to mine. Inside I cried. Someone I love so much can only be called mine on a silly #2 lead pencil.

January, 1992

Today there was a message from Kenny's birth mother on my machine. She wanted him to call her. We haven't seen her in over a year. I helped him dial her number. Then I leave the room. He's only seven and maybe he needs me when he talks with her, but I can't handle it. I pace the floor, far enough away that I won't be tempted to overhear their conversation.

April, 1992

Today Kenny's mother calls me. She's been really sick since before the holidays and has been hospitalized twice. She sounds weak and scared. I can hear the fear in her voice for the first time in all the years we've known each other. Her usual optimism is gone. Her brother is near death from this too, and her sister is becoming symptomatic. I guess they all shared needles, but she's never actually told me that. She tells me she's lost all the weight she'd gained for a while, and her body has become a stranger. That seems to upset her the most. She asks how Kenny is doing, and I say fine. We always lie to each other about him, because it helps each of us to feel better. She asks to see him again . . . why do I think she means for one last time? We make the visit arrangements.

I ask her to have someone call me if things get bad for her and she can't call herself. She agrees.

June, 1992

No one called me. But in the paper I find a death notice for Kenny's birth mother. I told him he didn't need to go to school, because we had an appointment. After the other kids left, I told him. He kept crying, "No, no, no." He's been with me for years, but he still loves her too. We cry together, me not only for her but because I'm more scared for Kenny now.

April, 1993

My little foster son died last week. Another foster parent who tried to support me in my suffering ran from the cemetery in tears. To reach my son's burial site, we had to walk by her little girl's grave. It's only been a month since we buried her together, and her mother couldn't take it. How will we all not only survive this silent war, but support each other as well?

May, 1993

Yesterday I got a letter from a very dear friend apologizing at great length for not knowing my son had died two weeks ago, therefore missing his funeral, when I had been there for her son's funeral three years ago. How can I be upset with her? It seems our extended circles of friends and families are all coming to know each other through the deaths of our loved ones from this disease.

Children orphaned by it move into new families who, by their very sensitivity to the disease, will only expose them to more death when other children in their care, other birth parents of these kids, and others in their circle continue to die.

Some people would trivialize the deaths of such kids and the impact those deaths make on the families caring for them. "You know that was a medically fragile child." "Oh, it was just your foster child who died, not one of your own?" Make no mistake: if we serve these children well, we bring them as much joy as possible, and mourn them greatly when they are gone. In no way do I regret my own work with any of these children. I only wish I had the power to do miracles for the sick ones, so that I wouldn't need to wish for the strength to help the well ones survive all this over, and over, and over.

For myself, I pray the Lord will give me strength of heart and a long enough time on this earth that my children will be grown before I die. Amen.

June, 1993

One of my adopted children hasn't expressed much emotion about the baby's death. In therapy, it comes out that his death conjures up memories of her birth mother's death, and the recent death of her little friend. She's not sure how to express her feelings and I'm sadly thinking that with all the loss she's experienced my kid should be a pro at crying. Except that over-whelming loss shuts her down. How will my kids come out of this epidemic? Will their bodies survive and their hearts die?

• • •

Two Women, One Future

There were two women who came to know each other, whose lives became entwined only because they both loved the same little boy.

The first woman was a Black woman who was dying. The other was a White woman who was a foster parent. In an in-creasingly polarized and segregated society, they were perhaps exceptions to the "norm." Because of their personal experiences, they were able to talk with each other.

When the Black woman gave birth to her son, she was home-less and voluntarily, though reluctantly, placed him in foster care. She was sick, and knew she couldn't care for both of them. Although she missed him, she was able to put his needs first. The agency charged with finding her son a home knew of the

White woman, and asked her to care for the little boy, who might also become ill like his mother. She agreed, and soon loved the little boy like her own.

For almost a year, the foster mother and the little boy heard nothing from the birth mother. Occasionally, the social worker reported that the mother's health was poor, and her housing situation uncertain. His mother wanted the little boy to stay with the foster mother so he could be well cared for.

Then one day, the social worker called and asked the foster mother if the little boy's mother and his brother and sister could come to visit. The foster mother was a little nervous about meeting them.

The foster mother baked cookies for them. The social worker brought them in her car and made introductions. When they sat down, the foster mother put the little boy on his mother's lap for the first time since he was born. He looked like her! The visit was both happy and sad for everyone. The mother was so thin and sick. Both mothers knew there wasn't much time left in this life, yet so much needed to be said. When the social worker took the mother and her other children back to their emergency housing, the mother cried all the way back: she was happy her little boy was loved, and was surprised that she was welcomed at his home.

Then, finally, a medication became available. The mother got it, and for the next few years her health stayed stable and she gained some weight. She continued to struggle with drugs, but finally succeeded. The two mothers came to know each other.

One day arrangements were made between them for one of the other children of the mother to visit for the weekend with the foster mother and his little brother. Both mothers had talked about his need for special care after his birth mother died. There were no suitable relatives.

He came for the visit, and never left. It was very hard on his birth mother to let him go: people criticized her for giving her son up. They said she gave him to White people and were angry with her. People were angry with the foster mother too: they said she "stole" a Black child from his race. But the two mothers loved the boys, and planned together for their future care. And the boys thrived and were happy.

As the birth mother got sicker, her other child—a girl—began to spend more time with the foster mother and her brothers. The mothers explained their relationship to each other as a friendship, and the children accepted this. Child welfare officials were leery of such a strange alliance.

By now, with the birth mother's blessing, both boys were adopted by the foster mother, and this brought her sadness, yet peace. Then one day the birth mother died. The boys and their only mother now went to her funeral. People they had never met were there. They met their father and his family. After the funeral, the girl stayed with the foster mother for a while, while her father tried to get life in order for them. But he couldn't do it. The foster mother loved the girl too, and the boys were happy to be with their sister. The foster mother asked the father if the older sister could stay with her. He loved the children, but knew he couldn't take care of them without the help of their mother. Together, the foster mother and father went to court, and made custody arrangements for the older sister. The foster mother and the father would share custody, and the sister would make her home with her younger brothers. But people on the street were cruel to the father; they said he had sold his children. It was very hard for him.

The children were happy to be reunited. Their father came each week at least for dinner, and sometimes stayed with them for a few days. They came to know their grandmother and aunt, who became relatives also to all the other children in the family.

There is a picture hanging up of the dead mother in the house to this day. She is never forgotten, and always loved. Flowers are placed on the altar at church by the children on holidays. Her braveness in being able to plan for her children, while trying to deal with her own impending death, will always be remembered.

Maybe the day will come when we can openly talk about why she died without fear, and how two women who were strangers became friends, held each other, cried together, and talked about a future only one of them would see.

"Ann"

Ann is a forty-year-old woman from a large Catholic family. She raises her two children, thirteen-year-old John and three-and-one-half-year-old Sara, in a home they own in a suburban community. Her husband Jack died of cancer and AIDS. Ann is also infected, but neither child is. She tells some of her story.

Learning to Live with HIV Disease

You know, for the week or two before we got the test results I was hoping and praying and saying, "OK, God, Jack's got it, I wish he didn't have it, but he's got it, but I'm going to be OK, my baby's going to be OK. Right? You can't give us a triple whammy here." And then when I got the news, it just hit me . . . and I remember going completely numb. There was a lot of disbelief, maybe some denial, and I wanted it to be a mistake. I wanted it to be an error in the lab, or whatever could explain it. I just wanted it to be wrong. And it wasn't wrong.

There are all those questions. How? When? Why? Where? Who? Well, we know how he got it, he slept with someone.

When? We don't know when. We assume it better have been before he married me, you know. Why? We'll never know why he got it. Where? Who? How do you answer that? I can't answer the questions. . . .

They say it's usually ten years after the infection you can start expecting problems. Well, I want to know if I'm going to be here to see my daughter make communion in four years. That's important to me. . . . And not knowing when this happened to Jack makes me a little crazy. If it happened before we got married, I married him in '86, I met him in '85, so here it is, '94, that's nine years. Does that mean next year is my D-day? I don't want to think like that.

After I had the ulcer attack in April, in June I had bronchial pneumonia, and then I got another bout of it in September. . . . I'm OK, you know. . . . It's very uncertain, because every time I don't feel well, I wonder, "Now what?" and that's the part I don't like living with. . . . I was never a sickly kind of a person. It's annoying, more than anything it's annoying. . . . Every little thing that happens I think, "Oh, is this it? Is this it?" And I'm not one to panic. I get migraine headaches and I think, oh it's a tumor. I saw it with Jack. He went from having a sinus infection to having this huge tumor in his head. . . . These are major things that I don't want to expect, I don't want to look forward to, I don't want to know about. And I'm mature enough to know that I have to have my eyes wide open, but I'm a coward. I don't want to know about it.

I wanted to be a nurse when I was younger. Then when I was in high school, I really wanted to be a teacher. I really wanted to work with children, in any capacity, social work, teaching, anything. And I only did two years of college and then I stopped, but I worked as a paraprofessional, I taught Sunday School. . . . But I always want to have more kids. . . . I do feel cheated. With Jack, I would have loved another one. But now I'm forty, and even if I met a man tomorrow and he wanted to get married next month, I probably would have chanced another one, but now I can't. That hurts. It hurts. There are days I go into a grand funk, and it stays for weeks.

I have yet to pursue going to an HIV support group. I have a fear about that. And it's not a fear like I'm going to catch something, it's a fear like, "I don't want to have to need them." . . . When the widows-with-children support group came about, when we lost our spouses to cancer, we all had something in common: the hospital bills, or running back and forth, getting babysitters, juggling this, juggling that, not taking care of yourself, and it really helped us. I'm sure an HIV support group would help too, but I'm almost afraid to become attached to these people. If I have to watch them die, then I'm gonna say, "Oh my God, is that gonna happen to me?" I would dwell on it a lot more than I do now. I don't know if I want to cross that line yet.

I wish for a lot. I wish that it didn't exist. I wish that I never heard of it. Part of me also wishes they never found it in Jack and I could be walking around deaf, dumb and blind about it. But I do know. I'm OK. I don't like it. I hate it. But I'm OK with it, because I choose to live with it. It may sound like a cliche, but I choose to live with it. I have a secret weapon. I have God. Every part of me believes that. That's my protection.

John, the Son

John's thirteen. He's happy because now he's an inch taller than me. . . . I was married once before to John's father, and when John was two, his father came home one day and announced that he didn't want to be married anymore. He didn't want any responsibility. So John and I were on our own. He hasn't seen his biological father since he was two and a half, and he's thirteen now. When John was four, I met Jack. And John got attached to him right away. When he knew we were getting married, he asked Jack one day, without me being in the room, "Can I call you Daddy?" and took Jack by surprise. He was the ring-bearer at our wedding. Jack adopted him. And now he's lost another father.

While Jack was sick, and he was home, John only knew about the cancer. . . . After Jack died, John slept on the couch in the living room for four and a half months. He was afraid to sleep downstairs in his bedroom. He was afraid to sleep at a friend's house, or be away from me for a day. He was afraid something was going to happen to me and Rachel.

A lot of people when Jack died said, "OK, John, you're the man of the house." "You got to take care of your mother." That was terrible. I mean, that weighs heavy on a kid, especially when they don't want to be bothered.

We've always been very attached, and now he's going through the thirteen-year-old-nasty-attitude-phase. . . . He had a very rough time in school last year. And even as angry as he can get at me, if I'm not feeling well I try not to emphasize it too much, but he'll say, "Are you all right? Are you all right? You better go to the doctor." He's gotten a little bit better about being away from me. I guess part of that's the age. But I don't think he could handle it. If he knew that I had it, and I was dealing with . . .

Even now, he's been to Yale with me when there's summer vacation. He knows I have to go there every three months. And he questioned it one time, and I said to him, "Well, John, it's sort of like a clinic. And because I don't have very good medical coverage and all, I get free checkups because, remember, I was anemic, and they were worried, and I don't want to get sick. They do blood work and it's all free." And he bought it. And he doesn't question it, and I'm very fortunate. 'Cause I don't lie.

You know, it's very hard for me to tell a lie to my son. But this is necessary, I feel.

I've questioned counselors, I've questioned the pastor, the old principal that we had, and they all agree, there's no reason to tell him. And believe me, there are times when he's driving me nuts, and I feel like the stress. . . . I mean, stress is very bad for this, and let's face it, my middle name is stress. And I want to say to him, "Do you know what you're doing to me? . . ." But I don't, because I don't want to use it as a weapon. I can't do that to a thirteen-year-old. I know he'll freak out. Because he'll think now that, "that's it, it's over," and I don't want him to give up his zest for life, or going through whatever he's supposed to go through for a thirteen-year-old. Goofin' off, or goofin' around, or whatever he's supposed to be doing, I don't want him to give that up.

I don't know when I would tell him. Sometimes I think about it and I'm scared. I don't think he would be afraid of hugging me or kissing me or anything like that. I think he would just be terrified of losing me. Terrified. If I have to, if I get seriously ill, . . . then I might tell him. But I keep hoping that the age will go higher and higher and higher, and he'll be more stable, and OK about it. I can't put the burden on him.

I had to make a will up after Jack died. Jack had asked my brother, "If anything happens to me or Ann, you've got to take care. . . ." No problem. But, I don't feel that comfortable with the decision now. Back then, it was "Thank you," at least somebody's around to pick up the pieces. But I don't feel that comfortable now. John isn't comfortable with it. And I say to myself, how could I *do* this to him? He wants to stay *here.*

We were on the waiting list for Big Brothers, and July will be two years we're on the waiting list. But now he's getting too old, at fourteen they cut it off. He needs a man around. He needs a mentor. You know, he's got a lot of buddies, friends, but he needs somebody to kind of take him under the wing, and unfortunately, family doesn't do that. Which is sad. I think it's like, "out of sight, out of mind." They don't pitch in, and that's been a big disappointment for me. Very big. I wish I could say my family is 100 percent but they're not. They're not. I have one brother . . . he has not been to my home since I told him. . . . I gave his wife all my maternity clothes. . . . I had a vision that she burned them.

John's a good student, but he doesn't push himself. I figure he's a solid B student. I want him to be on an honor roll before he gets out of eighth grade, just one time . . . but he leaves everything until the last minute. He's so typical. I've asked around with other parents of kids his age in his class, and he does OK, but he *could* do, the best. And I wish I could instill that in him. I've been trying to get him to have more independence, more responsibility, take more pride. You know, it's

like, I've got to get this job done, you know, and if I lay the
foundation, you know, then I don't have to worry.

Sara, the Daughter

Sara is three and a half and in September starts school three
mornings a week. . . . With Sara . . . now I'm very happy,
because she does have a normal life, and she is a handful, she's
wonderful, God bless her. And He did. I thought about that,
when I enroll her in school, if she still had had it [tested HIV
positive], I'd have to disclose that and I'd have been terrified of
her being ostracized. There's always gonna be one person that's
gonna spill the beans to the wrong person. And it's gonna be
like wild fire, it's gonna just spread.

Stigma

I think there's a lot of shame attached. And I can tell you, my
husband's glad that he died from cancer, and not the other. I
know if I have to die at any point, I don't want to die from that.
Why should I feel that kind of shame? But it's not for me. I don't
want people treating my memory, or my children, adversely. . . .
I don't want anyone to push away, back away, or cause any
problems. . . . You hear people talk. Even neighbors will say,
"Well thank God, can you imagine if it was AIDS?" And I think,
would you still come into my house and have a cup of coffee?
. . . I think if anyone backed off from me, it would crush me.

Isn't it funny how gays have to come out of the closet? Now
people with diseases have to come out of the closet. I mean,
cancer is a very serious illness. Diabetes. Heart disease. And
people aren't afraid of touching or being near these people. Let's
face it, cancer patients with the treatment, I mean, I saw Jack,
they can look pretty disgusting. And people are never afraid,
well why would you be afraid? . . . I wish I did have the courage
to stand up in the middle of somewhere and say, "Hey, I slept
with my husband. That's how *I* got it."

People in the media, the celebrities that succumb to it . . .
they're in a different category. They're respected, they're brave,
they're courageous. Why aren't I? I mean, I think I am, but I
don't look to get that adulation, it's not part of the deal. I just
want to be healthy.

I wish people could be a little more kind and understanding,
and compassionate. How do you enlighten people? They tell
you in so many ways you can only get this by intercourse and
by sharing a needle. Well, I'm not going to do that to people
who walk into my home. What is it about that that people don't
believe or understand? It's pretty simple language. It's pretty
basic. What is wrong?

Taking Care of My Family

Jack's cousin is a priest, and I did tell him. . . . And he called me around the holidays, and I said I feel like I should be doing more. And he said, Ann, you're doing exactly what you're supposed to be doing now, which is you're taking care of you, and you're taking care of your children, and that's a big job, don't minimize it. And it kind of put it into perspective. And I don't take very good care of myself. I got a lot of dark circles under my eyes, I need more rest, and I could use a helping hand. But he was right. I have a family. They come first. We come first. Does that make me selfish? I was feeling that way. . . .

I don't want to lose the house. I've talked to the lawyers. I've talked to a financial lady. I pay my mortgage, but should I put it in somebody's name? So that if I get ill, and I run out of insurance and I have to apply for Medicaid, they won't tell me, "Sell the house." I couldn't fathom doing that, that's so unfair. That the government would . . . make me get rid of my stability here? This is home! . . . I can't imagine in the United States of America anyone going without food, without a place to live, and without medical care. I don't care if you're a Donald Trump, or if you live on the street, I can't imagine anybody being denied those three basic things. . . . It's scary. I don't want to have to lose what I have. So I'll just try to have to stay healthy. It's just sheer will.

My doctor told me we won't see a cure in this lifetime. I looked at him and I said, "How can you be so negative?" . . . I don't live every day as if it's my last day. . . . I don't choose to think that I'm dying. Even if I had cancer, even if they told me I had cancer tomorrow, I'd probably thumb my nose up at it because I'd say, fine, you can treat it, get rid of it, just leave me alone. I have a job to do here. And my job is to raise my family. Whether it's alone, or not. But I refuse to let my children be raised by anybody else. I'm the only mother I want them ever to know, or need. I don't care who in the family . . . I don't want anybody to raise my children. That's what *I* was chosen for.

Epilogue

Women and Children in a Time of Plague in America

ALVIN NOVICK

A woman infected by HIV, insofar as we currently know, almost invariably progresses to AIDS, serious illness, and death over a period of about ten to fifteen years from her initial infection. All of the children of women infected by HIV will experience, at the very least, loss of their mother, and perhaps their father and one or more siblings during their childhood. Who are these women and children? What are the children's needs?

In the United States today, about 80 percent of the women who are infected by HIV are African-American or Latina. Most of these women are poor. Many live in neighborhoods in our inner cities. Many women infected by HIV are single mothers. Some are in durable or temporary relationships with men, not necessarily the men by whom they were infected. A high proportion of these mothers have lives disrupted by deep poverty, drug or alcohol use, teenage motherhood, petty crime, imprisonment, unstable living situations, and limited education and job skills. Many lack even a vision of how to improve or stabilize their lives and the lives of their children.

In this context, they face their own deteriorating health and the demands of establishing and maintaining ties to health care for themselves, possibly for one or more of their children, and sometimes for their spouse or partner. A nuclear family may have three or more members who are infected, ill, dying, or already dead, and one or more members who are well but, as we say, "affected" by AIDS.

The household, if there is a stable context, is afflicted by worry and anticipation of life threatening illness, future transmissions, confusing and demanding health care, and then by disabling illness and death. The family risks being severely stigmatized by neighbors, extended family members, or others in the community.

Mothers and their children will often exhibit self-isolation (from depression, guilt, or fear of rejection), low self-image, defiance or anger, denial, and confusion. These characteristics will emerge and recede from time to time and make for a troubled and depleted household. In addition, these negative emotions in the mother will generate a range of consequences in the affected children. Some families will have the inner strength and outside support to weather these challenges. Many will not.

Many affected families, including the affected children, will experience a "loss of the future." That is, the future may come to seem too bleak, too hopeless to plan for, too unsolvable to be real. Many affected families—perhaps most—will lose the past. They will lose the ties to their past that the dead mother, father, or siblings represent. If the dead are seen as seriously contaminated, stigmatized, or "bad," family members may lose not only their physical presence but also good memories and supportive stories about their lives. Many children will float day to day unless they receive wise and informed counsel and support.

Children, of course, depend for their development on socialization with family, schoolmates, teachers, other adult role models, and friends. If this socialization process is truncated or erased completely, affected children will be in need of experienced assistance if they are to grow into and occupy "life."

The troublesome and alarming concern is that many of the children affected by AIDS have poor access to the resources they need because of poverty, community disruption, minority status, or familial substance abuse. Before AIDS, we had already abandoned many of these children to constricted and narrow fates. Have we failed to notice that they have the cards unreasonably stacked against them? The epidemic of psychological disability that has engulfed large numbers of our minority, inner-city youths since at least the 1950s has been noticed with horror, but without either substantial scholarship or, on the whole, rational, well-reasoned supportive services.

What will the children affected by AIDS need?

History and comparison with other plagues chiefly teach us that these children will need sensitive and decent care in orphanhood—stability, love, safety, and understanding. The modes of orphan care and services have, of course, improved since earlier plagues. But many of these orphans will be children of color and of poverty. They will have special needs.

These children will need help when their mothers and siblings are ill and dying—to understand what is happening and why, to ease the physical burdens of taking on adult tasks, and to anchor them to a secure future. Then they will require tender care to restore their futures, assuage their fears, relieve the futility of their lives, bolster their self-images, and foster their ability to develop visions and to reach toward those visions. To do those things, we need to know them and for them to know "us"—the restorers.

Who will provide such care? We cannot discern any positive lessons from the past beyond the material care of orphans. The other lesson from the past is that these services were not developed. Nor have they been for the AIDS-unaffected children of our inner-city ghettos.

Can the needs of AIDS-affected children compete with the needs of all of the other children with whom they share their communities? Probably not. Thus, we may have to take a broader brush and commit resources to the vast, demanding, and deeply worthy task of restoring the lives and the futures of all of our neglected and forlorn children—and their parents and neighbors.

Clearly we need the scholarly evaluation of a broad range of social scientists. We need to examine the children and the range of their settings and to describe their depletions, their resilience, their obstacles, and their resources. We need to assess the competence, authority, and scope of supportive services, if any. We need support for pilot projects, model programs, and the ability to showcase and clone some of that work.

Who will speak for these children? Who, indeed? If we look at other plagues, perhaps no one, or no one with the clout to serve them well. Kindly bureaucracies will surely try to arrange foster care with family members or with strangers and will sometimes be able to arrange adoption. Group homes and orphanages will be developed, and they may come to be administered in a user-friendly way. What will continuing stigmatization do to affect these settings? Will the children be pitied and patronized, or loved and nurtured? Will we know what is happening to them? Will we care?

Resource Guide

This guide lists books, articles, videos, national organizations, and state and local programs that can assist professionals, parents, and policy-makers who are trying to help children and youths living with AIDS in their families and communities. It is far from exhaustive but provides easy access to some key sources (though phone numbers and addresses may change). To keep abreast of new developments in the literature, in video, and in organizations providing services, two additional research tools merit special mention:

National AIDS Clearinghouse
Department of Health and Human Services, Public Health Service
P.O. Box 6003, Rockville, MD 20849-6003
(800) 458-5231   (800) 243-7012 (TDD/Deaf Access)

The clearinghouse provides helpful information on HIV/AIDS service organizations, educational materials, and funding sources. Reference specialists will run free computer searches of four key databases: (a) *Resources and services*—descriptions of more than sixteen thousand organizations that provide AIDS-related prevention, education, and social services; (b) *Educational materials*—more than nine thousand descriptions of books, videos, reports, brochures, directories, etc.; (c) *Funding*—lists of HIV-related funding opportunities, including application processes and deadlines; (d) *AIDS school health education*—descriptions of educational resources for professionals. The search printouts that you receive include, for each item found, key descriptive information, including all information necessary to find, purchase, or borrow the item.

National Library of Medicine, MEDLARS System

NLM maintains a number of AIDS-related databases that can be searched at libraries and other institutions, and through personal computers. GRATEFUL MED is an inexpensive NLM microcomputer-based software package that provides access to more than twenty databases in the MEDLARS system. It is available for IBM/compatible and Apple computers. The primary AIDS-related databases are AIDSLINE (thousands of literature references published since 1980, 50 percent with abstracts, updated weekly); AIDSTRIALS and AIDSDRUGS (information about clinical trials); DIRLINE (annotated directory of more than seventeen thousand organizations, more than eleven hundred of which provide AIDS-related services); AVLINE (audiovisual teaching packages, more than one hundred of them AIDS related); BIOETHICSLINE (published bioethical information); and POPLINE (population information resources). NLM also produces a monthly bibliography of articles, videos, conference papers, etc. Phone numbers for further information:

AIDSLINE and accessing NLM databases: (800) 638-8480

AIDS Bibliography (and general AIDS reference questions): (800) 272-4787

Bibliography

General Background on the Pandemic

Books

Cohen, F., and J. Durham, eds. 1993. *Women, children, and HIV/AIDS.* New York: Springer.

DiClemente, R., ed. 1992. *Adolescents and AIDS: A generation in jeopardy.* Newbury Park, Calif.: Sage.

Fee, E., and D. Fox. 1988. *AIDS: The burdens of history.* Berkeley: University of California Press.

Kaplan, E., and M. Brandeau, eds. 1994. *Modeling the AIDS epidemic: Planning, policy, and prediction.* New York: Raven.

Kurth, A., ed. 1993. *Until the cure: Caring for women with HIV.* New Haven: Yale University Press.

Levine, C., ed. 1993. *A death in the family: Orphans of the HIV epidemic.* New York: United Hospital Fund.

Levine, C., and G. Stein, eds. 1994. *Orphans of the HIV epidemic: Unmet needs in six U.S. cities.* New York: United Hospital Fund.

Mack, A., ed. 1991. *In time of plague: The history and social consequences of lethal epidemic disease.* New York: New York University Press.

Mann, J., D. Tarantola, and T. Netter, eds. 1992. *A global report: AIDS in the world.* Cambridge: Harvard University Press.

National Commission on AIDS. 1993. *AIDS: An expanding tragedy.* Washington, D.C.: National Commission on AIDS. Other Commission reports of interest include: *The challenge of HIV/AIDS in communities of color* (December, 1992); *Preventing AIDS in adolescents* (June, 1993). Commission Reports can be obtained through the National AIDS Clearinghouse, (800) 458-5231.

National Research Council, Panel on Monitoring the Social Impact of the AIDS Epidemic. 1993. *The social impact of AIDS in the United States.* Washington, D.C.: National Academy Press.

Pizzo, P. A., and C. M. Wilfert, eds. 1994. *Pediatric AIDS: The challenge of HIV infection in infants, children and adolescents.* 2d ed. Baltimore: Williams and Wilkins. This multiauthored text contains chapters dealing with the epidemiologic, clinical, psychological, social and political aspects of pediatric AIDS. It is currently the definitive work on the subject. Table 43.1 lists some summer camps available to families living with HIV.

Sills, Y. G. 1994. *The AIDS pandemic: Social perspectives.* Westport, Conn.: Greenwood.

Sontag, S. 1988. *AIDS and its metaphors.* New York: Farrar, Straus, Giroux.

Stine, G. 1993. *Acquired immune deficiency syndrome: Biological, medical, social and legal issues.* Englewood Cliffs, N.J.: Prentice Hall.

Stuber, M., ed. 1992. *Children and AIDS.* Washington, D.C.: American Psychiatric Press.

United National Children's Fund. 1993. *AIDS: The second decade: A focus on youth and women.* New York: UNICEF.

Monographs, Chapters, and Articles

Black, M. 1991. *AIDS and orphans in Africa.* New York: UNICEF.

Bonuck, K. A. 1993. AIDS and families: Cultural, psychosocial, and functional impacts. *Social Work in Health Care* 18 (2): 75–89.

Conover, T. 1994. The hand-off: Christy picks a mother. *The New York Times Magazine,* May 8, 1994.

HIV and street youth. 1992. Special issue of *AIDS Education and Prevention.*

Hunter, S. 1990. Orphans as a window on the AIDS epidemic in sub-Saharan Africa: Initial results and implications of a study in Uganda. *Social Science and Medicine* 51 (6): 681–690.

Michaels, D., and C. Levine. 1992. Estimates of the number of motherless youth orphaned by AIDS in the United States. *Journal of the American Medical Association* 268 (24): 3456–3461.

Nicholas, S., and E. Abrams. 1992. The "silent" legacy of AIDS: Children who survive their parents and siblings. *Journal of the American Medical Association* 268 (24): 3478–3479.

Preble, E. A. 1990. The impact of HIV/AIDS on African children. *Social Science and Medicine* 31 (6): 671–680.

World Health Organization Global Programme on AIDS. 1991. *The care and support of children of HIV-infected parents.* New York: WHO.

Stigma and Its Effect on the Family

Birenbaum, A. 1970. On managing a courtesy stigma. *Journal of Health and Social Behavior* 11: 196–206.

Gallo, A. M., et al. 1991. Stigma in childhood chronic illness: A well sibling perspective. *Pediatric Nursing* 17: 21–25.

Goffman, E. 1963. *Stigma: Notes on management of spoiled identity.* Englewood Cliffs, N.J.: Prentice Hall.

Lipson, M. 1993. Disclosure within families. *AIDS Clinical Care* 5 (6): 43–47.

Powell-Cope, G., and M. Brown. 1992. Going public as an AIDS family caregiver. *Social Science and Medicine* 34 (5): 571–580.

Child and Family Response and Coping

Ahmed, Paul, ed. 1992. *Living and dying with AIDS.* New York: Plenum Press.

Barth, R., J. Pietrzak, and M. Ramler. 1993. *Families living with drugs and HIV: Intervention and treatment.* New York: Guilford.

Bauman, L., and L. Wiener, eds. 1994. *Journal of Developmental and Behavioral Pediatrics* 15 (3). June supplement. The supplement's fourteen articles provide an overview of research about the psychological and social impacts of the AIDS epidemic on children and families. Contains comprehensive bibliographies and presents research recommendations.

Berlinsky, E. B., and H. B. Biller. 1982. *Parental death and psychological development.* Lexington, Mass.: Lexington.

Bor, R., R. Miller, and E. Goldman. 1993. HIV/AIDS and the family: A review of research in the first decade. *Journal of Family Therapy* 15: 187–204.

Bowlby, J. 1969. *Attachment and loss.* Vols. 1 and 2. New York: Basic.

Boyd-Franklin, N., G. Steiner, and M. Boland, eds. 1994. *Children, families, and HIV/AIDS.* New York: Guilford.

Bridge, P., A. F. Mirsky, and F. K. Goodwin, vol. eds. 1988. Psychological, neuropsychiatric, and substance abuse aspects of AIDS. In *Advances in Biochemical Psychopharmacology.* Vol. 44. New York: Raven.

Brown, M. A., and G. M. Powell-Cope. 1991. AIDS family caregiving: Transitions through uncertainty. *Nursing Research* 40 (6): 338–345.

Coles, Robert. 1990. *The spiritual life of children.* Boston: Houghton Mifflin.

Conviser, R. 1991. *Caring for families with HIV: Case studies of pediatric HIV/AIDS demonstration projects.* Newark, N.J.: National Pediatric HIV Resource Center.

Dane, B., and S. O. Miller. 1992. *AIDS: Intervening with hidden grievers.* Westport, Conn.: Auburn House.

Doka, K. 1980. *Disenfranchised grief: Recognizing hidden sorrow.* Lexington, Mass.: Lexington.

Draimin, B., J. Hudis, and J. Segura. 1992. *The mental health needs of well adolescents in families with AIDS.* New York: New York City Human Resources Administration, Division of AIDS Services.

Duffy, V. 1994. Crisis points in HIV disease. *AIDS Patient Care,* February, 28–32.

Edelman, H. 1994. *Motherless daughters: The legacy of loss.* Reading, Mass.: Addison Wesley.

Essa, E., and C. Murray. 1994. Research in review: Young children's understanding and experience with death. *Young Children,* May, 74–81. Includes useful bibliography.

Evans, M., et al. 1994. Counseling HIV-negative children of parents with HIV disease: A structured protocol. *AIDS Patient Care,* February, 16–19.

Feeman, D. J., and J. W. Hagen. 1990. Effects of childhood chronic illness on families. *Social Work in Health Care* 14: 37–53.

Furman, E. 1974. *A child's parent dies: Studies in childhood bereavement.* New Haven: Yale University Press.

Lipson, M. 1993. What do you say to a child with AIDS? *Hastings Center Report* 23 (2): 6–12.

Ostrow, D. G., and R. C. Kessler, eds. 1993. *Methodological issues in AIDS behavioral research.* New York: Plenum.

Rosen, H. 1985. *Unspoken grief: Coping with childhood sibling loss.* Lexington, Mass.: Lexington.

Schilling, R., et al. 1992. Bereavement groups for inner-city children. *Research on Social Work Practice* 3 (2): 405–419. Includes useful bibliography.

Winiarski, M. 1991. *AIDS-related psychotherapy.* New York: Pergamon.

Zambelli, G., and A. DeRosa. 1992. Bereavement support groups for school-age children: Theory, intervention, and case example. *American Journal of Orthopsychiatry* 62 (4): 484–493.

Child Welfare, Social Services, Education

Anderson, G., ed. 1990. *Courage to care: Responding to the crisis of children with AIDS.* Washington, D.C.: Child Welfare League of America. Has extensive resource guide and bibliography.

Barbour, R. S. 1994. Impact of working with people with HIV/AIDS: A review of the literature. *Social Science and Medicine* 39 (2): 221–232.

Behrman, R., ed. 1992. *School linked services: The future of children* 2 (1). Los Altos, Calif.: The David and Lucille Packard Foundation.

Child Welfare League of America. 1994. *Kinship care: A natural bridge.* Washington, D.C.: Child Welfare League of America.

Elster, A., and N. Kuznets. 1994. *AMA guidelines for adolescent preventive services (GAPS): Recommendations and rationale.* Baltimore: Williams and Wilkins.

General Accounting Office. 1990. *AIDS education: Programs for out-of-school youth slowly evolving.* Washington, D.C.: Superintendent of Documents.

Lynch, V., G. Lloyd, and M. Fimbres. 1993. *The changing face of AIDS: Implications for social work practice.* Westport, Conn.: Auburn House.

McCormack, T. 1990. *The AIDS benefit handbook: Everything you need to know about social security, welfare, Medicaid, Medicare, food stamps, drugs and other benefits.* New Haven: Yale University Press.

Morales, J., and M. Bok. 1992. *Multicultural human services for AIDS treatment and prevention.* Binghamton, N.Y.: Haworth.

National Hispanic Education and Communications Projects (HDI). 1990. *Latina AIDS action plan and resource guide.* Washington, D.C.: HDI Projects.

Samuels, S. E., and M. Smith. 1993. *Condoms in the schools.* Menlo Park, Calif.: Henry Kaiser Family Foundation.

School-Based Adolescent Health Care Program. 1993. *The answer is at school: Bringing health care to our students.* Washington, D.C.: Robert Wood Johnson Foundation.

Schulman, I., and R. Behrman, eds. 1993. *Adoption: The future of children* 3 (1). Los Altos, Calif.: The David and Lucille Packard Foundation.

Legal Resources

Albert, P., et al. 1992. *AIDS practice manual.* New York: National Lawyer's Guild AIDS Network.

Burris, S., H. Dalton, and J. Miller, eds. 1993. *AIDS law today: A new guide to the public.* New Haven: Yale University Press.

English, A. 1992. The HIV-AIDS epidemic and the child welfare system: Protecting the rights of infants, young children, and adolescents. *Iowa Law Review* 77 (4): 1509–1560.

Feldesman, T., et al. 1992. *Legal issues in pediatric HIV practice: A handbook for health care providers.* Newark, N.J.: National Pediatric HIV Resource Center.

Haralambie, A. M. 1993. *The child's attorney: A guide to representing children in custody, adoption, and protection cases.* Chicago: American Bar Association.

Holder, A. 1985. *Legal issues in pediatrics and adolescent medicine.* New Haven: Yale University Press.

Horowitz, R. M., and H. A. Davidson. 1984. *Legal rights of children.* Colorado Springs: Shepard's/McGraw Hill. With supplements.

Hunter, N., and W. Rubenstein, eds. 1992. *The AIDS agenda: Emerging issues in civil rights.* New York: The New Press.

Rennert, S. 1989. *AIDS and persons with developmental disabilities.* Washington, D.C.: American Bar Association.

Soler, M., et al. 1989. *Representing the child client.* New York: Matthew Bender.

Children's Books

* specifically discusses AIDS

Boulden, J. 1992. *Uncle Jerry has AIDS.* Weaverville, Calif.: Boulden Publishing (P.O. Box 1186, Weaverville, CA 96093. [800] 238-8433 or [707] 538-3797). In English and Spanish.*

———. 1989. *Saying goodbye bereavement activity book.* Weaverville, Calif.: Boulden Publishing.

Clifton, L. 1983. *Everett Anderson's goodbye.* New York: Holt, Rinehart and Winston. Boy experiences death of his father.

dePaola, T. 1973. *Nana upstairs & Nana downstairs.* New York: G. P. Putnam's Sons. Explains death of great-grandmother to very young children.

Girard, L. 1991. *Alex, the kid with AIDS.* Morton Grove, Ill.: Albert Whitman and Co.*

Hausheer, R. 1989. *Children and the AIDS virus: A book for children, parents, & teachers.* New York: Clarion. Includes resource list and short bibliography.*

Hazen, B. 1985. *Why did Grandpa die?* New York: Golden.

Heegaard, M. 1991. *When someone has a very serious illness.* Minneapolis: Woodland. Many pages have room for children to draw pictures in response to text.

Hickman, M. 1983. *Last week my brother Anthony died.* Nashville: Abingdon.

Jordan, M. 1989. *Losing Uncle Tim.* Morton Grove, Ill.: Albert Whitman and Co. Death of favorite uncle to AIDS.*

Kliman, G. 1993. *My personal life history book: A guided activity workbook for foster children, their families, caseworkers, and teachers.* Available from Gilbert Kliman, M.D., Director, The Children's Psychological Trauma Center, 2105 Divisidero, San Francisco, CA 94115. See Chapter 7 for description.

Kohlenberg, S. 1993. *Sammy's mommy has cancer.* Magination.

Kubler-Ross, E. 1982. *Remember the secret.* Berkeley, Calif.: Celestial Arts.

Merrifield, M. 1990. *Come sit by me.* Toronto: Women's Press. Schoolmate with AIDS.*

Mills, J. 1993. *Gentle willow: A story for children about dying.* Magination.

Mollel, T. 1990. *The orphan boy.* New York: Clarion.

Penn, A. 1993. *The kissing hand.* Washington, D.C.: Child Welfare League of America. Helps children cope with separations of all types.

Pollack, E. 1992. *Whisper whisper Jesse, whisper whisper Josh: A story about AIDS.* Cambridge, Mass.: Advantage/Aurora. Superb discussion of secrecy about AIDS.*

Prestine, J. 1993. *Someone special died.* Carthage, Ill.: Fearon Teacher Aids, Paramount Communications Co.

Sanford, D. 1989. *David has AIDS.* Portland, Ore.: Multnomah. Religious beliefs of hemophiliac boy with AIDS help child and family cope with death.*

Schilling, S., and J. Swain. 1989. *My name is Jonathan (and I have AIDS).* Denver: Prickly Pair.*

Sendzik, D. 1993. *Josie's story.* New York: Metropolitan Community Church of New York. English and Spanish version coloring book tells story of child whose mother is HIV-infected.*

Simor, N. 1986. *The saddest time.* Niles, Ill.: Albert Whitman. Stories of deaths of uncle, classmate, and grandmother, with children's reactions.

Starkman, N. 1988. *Z's gift.* Seattle: Comprehensive Health Education Foundation. Child's empathy toward schoolteacher with AIDS.*

Tasker, M. 1992. *Jimmy and his family.* Bethesda, Md.: Association for the Care of Children's Health. Child's first-person account in English and Spanish of what it is like to live with HIV disease; depicts love and family support.*

————. 1988. *Jimmy and the eggs virus.* Newark, N.J.: National Pediatric HIV Resource Center. Child's perspective on learning about being HIV infected.*

Verniero, J. 1994. *You can call me Willy: A story to help children learn about AIDS.* New York: Brunner/Mazel. For children ages four to eight.*

Viorst, J. 1971. *The tenth good thing about Barney.* New York: Atheneum. Boy mourning death of cat and remembering good things to tell at cat's funeral, including the tenth, that the cat will nourish new life.

Walker, A. W. 1967. *To hell with dying.* New York: Harcourt Brace Jovanovich.

White, E. B. 1952. *Charlotte's web.* New York: Harper and Row.

Wiener, L., A. Best, and P. A. Pizzo. 1994. *Be a friend: Children who live with HIV speak.* Morton Grove, Ill.: Albert Whitman and Co. Art and writing of children who live with HIV.*

Williams, M. 1971. *The velveteen rabbit.* Garden City, N.J.: Doubleday.

Zolotow, C. 1974. *My grandson Lew.* New York: Harper and Row. Child recalls memories of grandfather who died when child was very young.

Books for Older Children and Teenagers

Baker, L. 1991. *You and HIV: A day at a time.* Philadelphia: W. B. Saunders. Describes HIV transmission, diagnosis, treatment, and emotional responses for children infected by HIV; useful also for affected siblings.

Blake, J. 1990. *Risky times, how to be AIDS-smart and stay healthy: A guide for teenagers.* New York: Workman. Has companion guide for parents.

Draimin, B. 1994. *Everything you need to know when a parent has AIDS.* New York: Rosen. For teens in grades 7–12.

————. 1993. *Coping when a parent has AIDS.* New York: Rosen. For teens who know or suspect a parent has AIDS; discusses siblings, deciding whom to tell, custody, hospital, saying goodbye, death, and starting anew.

Durant, P. 1992. *When heroes die.* New York: Atheneum. Hero-uncle with AIDS helps 12-year-old cope.

Grollman, E. 1993. *Straight talk about death for teenagers: How to cope with losing someone you love.* Boston: Beacon. Discusses AIDS in several sections.

Heegaard, M. 1990. *Coping with death & grief.* Minneapolis: Lerner. Shared accounts by young people of experiences with death.

Hein, K., and T. Foy. 1993. *AIDS: Trading fears for facts.* Fairfield, Ohio: Consumer Reports Books.

Krementz, J. 1981. *How it feels when a parent dies.* New York: Knopf. Personal accounts of youths 7–16 years old.

Richter, E. 1986. *Losing someone you love.* New York: G. P. Putnam's Sons. Personal accounts of youths who have experienced sibling death.

Rofes, E. 1985. *The kid's book about death and dying.* Boston: Little Brown. Written by and for youths.

White, R., and A. Cunningham. 1991. *Ryan White: My own story.* New York: Dial. Autobiography of youth with AIDS; especially useful for teens.

Books for Parents and Professionals

Bernstein, J. 1983. *Books to help children cope with separation and loss.* New York: R. R. Bowker. Bibliographic guide to fiction and nonfiction work for children ages 3–16.

Fassler, J. 1978. *Helping children cope.* New York: Free Press.

Jackson, E. 1965. *Telling a child about death.* New York: Channel. Discusses importance of honesty in answering children's questions.

Kubler-Ross, E. 1983. *On children and death.* New York: Macmillan. Describes how parents and children can and do cope with death; extensive bibliography, including books for children.

LeShan, E. 1976. *Learning to say goodbye.* New York: Macmillan. Discusses child's stages of mourning, fears, and fantasies after a parent has died.

Lightner, C., and N. Hathaway. 1990. *Giving sorrow words.* New York: Warner. Composite of many interviews with persons whose lives were changed by death.

Prestine, J. 1993. *Helping children cope with death: A practical resource guide.* Carthage, Ill.: Fearon Teacher Aids, Paramount Communications Company. Companion to *Someone special died;* includes suggested activities and excellent bibliography.

Schaefer, D., and C. Lyons. 1988. *How do we tell the children? Helping children understand and cope when someone dies.* Rev. ed. New York: Newmarket.

Stein, S. 1974. *About dying.* New York: Walker and Company. Separate text for children and adults on each page; child's story concerns death of grandfather and of bird.

Tasker, M. 1992. *How can I tell you? Secrecy and disclosure with children when a family member has AIDS.* Bethesda, Md.: Association for the Care of Children's Health. Excellent monograph discussing whether or not to tell about HIV diagnosis of parent or child; discusses discrimination, fears that child will tell others, unpredictable nature of child's response; includes personal stories and advice on phases of telling.

Tatelbaum, J. 1980. *The courage to grieve.* New York: Lippincott and Crowell. Includes advice about children's grief.

Videos

Videos about AIDS are produced for different audiences and with different purposes. No single source exists from which a consolidated and current listing of titles can be obtained. Perhaps the most useful way to obtain a printout of many titles is to call the National AIDS Clearinghouse's Educational Materials Database, (800) 458-5231. Three additional resources are: KIDSNET, a periodic listing by the National Association of Broadcasters of audio and video productions for kids, including several on AIDS, (202) 429-5447; National Adoption Information Clearinghouse, which produces a periodic catalog of audio-visual materials on adoption, (301) 231-6512; and Select

Media, Inc., which distributes film, video, and videodisc programs on HIV targeted to Latino and African-American youths, (212) 727-7507.

Mommy, who'll take care of me? is the hourlong video that inspired this book. It presents portraits of families facing AIDS through the eyes of the children. It also highlights some programs and services targeted to affected children and their families. Produced by and available from Connecticut Public Television, Hartford, Conn., (203) 278-5310.

The videos listed below are selected from the many found as this book was in its development. Many focus on educational and prevention efforts directed at elementary and high school students; others document the lives of persons living with HIV disease. We list these titles without recommendations, for we have not viewed each one.

AIDS: A challenge for the ministry. 1991. Video presents interviews with priests, staff, and parishioners from Episcopal churches in Philadelphia to examine the role of the church in dealing with AIDS. Available from Episcopal Community Services, Philadelphia, (215) 351-1458.

AIDS: A video primer for children. 1991. Fifteen-minute video provides information about AIDS and is structured to allow parents to interact with their children while viewing. Produced by and available from Berrent Publications, Roslyn, N.Y., (516) 365-4040.

Between friends. 1991. Twenty-six minutes, target age: junior and senior high school students. Spanish and English versions. Docudrama involving two girls, one of whom has a mother infected with HIV and who makes some bad choices about her own sexual behavior. Produced by the San Francisco Department of Health and available through the San Francisco Study Center, (800) 484-4173, ext. 1073.

Changing focus: Women, children and AIDS. 1990. Thirty-minute video focuses on increasing infections among women and increasing number of children orphaned. Uses interviews with two women to illustrate the effects of AIDS outside big cities and its impact on their children. Available from University of Wisconsin–Green Bay, (414) 465-2599.

Come sit by me: AIDS education. 1993. Eight minutes, target age: preschool and elementary school–aged children. Video is based on the children's book of the same name, in which a preschool child makes friends with a child who has AIDS. Available from AIMS Media, Chatsworth, Calif., (800) 367-2467.

A conversation with Magic. 1992. Thirty-minute video, originally broadcast as a Nickelodeon television special, features discussions with Magic Johnson about HIV disease. Available from the Magic Johnson Foundation, Los Angeles, (310) 785-0201.

The cool cat's show: HIV and AIDS. 1993. Twenty-one minutes, target age: elementary school children. Video presents information about HIV disease and how to prevent infection. Produced by and available from Children's Animated Television, Norwood, Mass., (617) 449-9699.

A day with Uncle Jerry. 1993. Seventeen minutes, target age: elementary school–aged children and their parents. Video presents information about HIV disease using animated characters and a story based on a visit of a child to her Uncle Jerry, who has AIDS. Available through Boulden Publishing, Weaverville, Calif., (800) 238-8433.

Double dutch–double jeopardy. 1992. Twenty-minute video features a double dutch champion and an HIV-infected AIDS educator who provide information about HIV. Cast includes singers, double dutchers, dancers, and drummers from many different racial and ethnic groups. Produced by Durrin Productions, Washington, D.C., (202) 387-6700.

Fighting for our lives: Women confronting AIDS. 1990. Twenty-nine-minute video presents ways in which women are becoming active in their own communities to reduce the spread of AIDS among women. Produced by the Center for Women's Policy Studies. Available from Women Make Movies, New York, (212) 925-0606.

Living with loss: Children and HIV. 1991. Twenty-minute video explores positive ways to cope with the death of a child to AIDS. Useful for siblings, caregivers, friends, and providers. Produced by and available from Child Welfare League of America, Washington, D.C., (908) 225-1900; (908) 417-0482, fax.

Sex education in America: AIDS and adolescents. 1993. Fifty-seven minutes, target age: adolescents. Video contains sexually explicit material and presents different health education programs in five communities. Produced by and available from Media Works, Boston, (800) 600-5779.

Special love. 1992. Eighteen-minute video addresses concerns of family members when a child is ill with cancer and explores the effects on siblings. Produced by and available from Modern Talking Picture Service, St. Petersburg, Fla., (800) 243-6877.

What if you give a kid a condom. 1992. Ten-minute video using rap and hip-hop music to present the dangers of unprotected sex. Produced by and available from the South Carolina AIDS Education Service, Columbia, S.C., (803) 736-1171.

National Organizations

This listing is not all-inclusive but highlights some key organizations that can provide information useful to HIV-affected children and their families.

AIDS Coordination Project
American Bar Association
1800 M St. NW
Washington, DC 20036
(202) 331-2248

AIDS Information Sourcebook
Oryx Press
4041 N. Central Ave., Suite 700

Phoenix, AZ 85012-3397
(800) 279-6799

AIDS Orphan Adoption Project
National Council for Adoption
1930 17th St. NW
Washington, DC 20009-6207
(800) 333-6232

The project operates the AIDS Orphan Adoption Exchange, which works with voluntary and public social service agencies to match waiting AIDS "orphans" with prospective adoptive parents. The project also conducts a media campaign to help educate the public about the AIDS orphan issue.

AIDS Policy Center
Intergovernmental Health Policy Project
2021 K St. NW, Suite 800
The George Washington University
Washington, DC 20006
(202) 872-1445

An excellent source for current AIDS-related legislation in each state.

Americans for a Sound AIDS Policy (ASAP)
Children's Assistance Fund
P.O. Box 17433
Washington, DC 20041-0433
(703) 471-7350   (703) 471-8409, fax

The fund was established to support children who are losing their parents to HIV disease. It provides emergency one-time financial assistance for necessities such as rent, utilities, groceries, telephone, and funeral expenses and counsels families who apply for such assistance about tapping into local networks that can provide such support. The fund operates a holiday gift program to provide presents for children in eligible families, helps to develop community resources to fill some of the gaps in the services available to these families, identifies families interested in providing foster care or adopting children orphaned by AIDS, and provides practical information to parents for planning the family's future (including legal, financial, and therapeutic support opportunities).

American Public Welfare Association
810 First St. NE, Suite 500
Washington, DC 20002-4267
(202) 682-0100   (202) 289-6555, fax

American School Health Association
7263 State Route 43
P.O. Box 708
Kent, OH 44240-0708
(216) 678-1601   (216) 678-4526

Association for the Care of Children's Health
7910 Woodmont Ave., Suite 300
Bethesda, MD 20814-3015
(301) 654-6549   (301) 986-4553, fax

The association's National Center for Family-Centered Care focuses on helping families of AIDS patients and infected children; Parent Network helps parents of children with special needs.

Child Welfare League of America
440 First St. NW, Suite 310
Washington, DC 20001-2085
(202) 638-2952   (202) 638-4004, fax

Produces standards, bibliographies, books, monographs, newsletters, videos etc. on foster care, adoption, family reunification, teen pregnancy, HIV.

Children's Defense Fund
25 E St. NW
Washington, DC 20001
(202) 628-8787

Center on Children and the Law
American Bar Association
1800 M St. NW, Suite 200S
Washington, DC 20036
(202) 331-2250   (202) 331-2225, fax

Compassionate Friends
P.O. Box 3696
Oak Brook, IL 60522-3696
(708) 990-0010   (708) 990-0246, fax

Nationwide self-help support group with 670 chapters for bereaved parents and siblings. Also produces brochures targeted at parents, brothers and sisters, stepfamilies, and grandparents.

Dougy Center
P.O. Box 86852
Portland, OR 97286
(503) 775-5683

Nonprofit center with nationwide affiliates for children who have lost a parent or sibling.

Grandparents United for Children's Rights
137 Larkin St.
Madison, WI 53705
(608) 238-8751

Advocacy group for grandparents acting as caregivers to their grandchildren.

Hispanic Designers, Inc.
National Hispanic Education and Communications Projects
1000 16th St. NW, Suite 401
Washington, DC 20036
(202) 452-8750   (202) 452-0086, fax

Specializes in Spanish/English education and information programs targeted to Hispanic community, with particular focus on women and twelve- to seventeen-year-old adolescents.

National AIDS Clearinghouse
Department of Health and Human Services, Public Health Service
P.O. Box 6003
Rockville, MD 20849-6003
(800) 458-5231   (800) 243-7012, TDD/Deaf Access

National AIDS Hotline
Centers for Disease Control and Prevention
(800) 342-AIDS, English
(800) 344-7432, Spanish
(800) 243-7889, TDD/Deaf Access

Twenty-four-hour, toll-free service that provides confidential information, referrals, and educational materials to the public.

National Center for Youth Law
114 Sansome St., Suite 900
San Francisco, CA 94104
(415) 543-3307   (415) 956-9024, fax

Provides advice, technical assistance, training, policy development in areas of law affecting poor children and adolescents. Publishes *Youth Law News*, an excellent overview of current developments in the law affecting these children.

National Institute of Mental Health, Office of AIDS Programs
Public Health Service, United States Department of Health and Human Services
Parklawn Bldg.

5600 Fishers Ln.
Rockville, MD 20857
(301) 443-7281

Provides information about current NIMH-funded research pertaining to affected children.

National Minority AIDS Council
300 I St. NE, Suite 400
Washington, DC 20002
(202) 544-1076

National Pediatric HIV Resource Center
Children's Hospital AIDS Program
Children's Hospital of New Jersey
15 S. Ninth St.
Newark, NJ 07107
(800) 362-0071   (201) 268-8251   (201) 485-2752, fax

Provides consultation, technical assistance, training, public policy guidance regarding children with HIV infection and their families and developing new programs to serve them; publishes monographs.

The Orphan Project
121 Avenue of the Americas, 6th Floor
New York, NY 10013
(212) 925-5290   (212) 925-5675, fax

The first education and policy center exploring policy options to meet the needs of all children affected by AIDS, with particular focus on issues of confidentiality and disclosure, custody and placement, benefits programs, and bereavement.

Sex Information and Education Council of the United States
130 W. 42d St., Suite 2500
New York, NY 10036-7901
(212) 819-9770   (212) 819-9776, fax

Education and policy center promoting education about sexuality and HIV. Publishes helpful bibliographies and booklets about sexuality education, HIV education and the AIDS epidemic, school condom distribution programs. Produces guide to AIDS videos.

State and Local Community Organizations

No list of state and local organizations serving children affected by HIV can be, or remain, complete: new organizations emerge and established organizations redefine their mission to meet the needs of affected children as well as infected family members. The easiest way to identify organizations in your community is to call the National AIDS Clearinghouse, listed above. Their computerized search can provide you with printouts describing all organizations in your area that might meet your needs. The following annotated listing is designed to give some sense of some of the services now being provided in different parts of the country for affected children. Some state health departments also can assist. For example, the New York State Department of Health's AIDS Institute now has staff hired specifically to work on AIDS "orphan" issues (212-613-2411). Note also some model program descriptions in Chapters 4 and 8 of this volume, and the resource directories in Levine's *A Death in the Family* (New York: United Hospital Fund, 1993), which lists New York City resources, and Kurth's *Until the Cure* (New Haven: Yale University Press, 1993), which focuses on programs helping women and their families.

Arizona

Arizona AIDS Project
4460 North Central Ave.
Phoenix, AZ 85012-1815
(602) 265-3300   (602) 265-9951, fax

The project's "Kids Central" programs include: Kid's Fun Day Party (monthly special fun event bringing together infected and affected children; volunteers provide transportation); JAY (Junior and Youth) Buddies and JAY Phone Buddies (after a training program, volunteer children and teens call others affected by AIDS); Children's Support Groups (grief counseling and a nutritional program). Project also provides legal clinics to help parents with custody planning. Motto: "Until there is a cure, there is care."

New Song Center for Grieving Children and Those Who Love Them
6947 E. McDonald Dr.
Paradise Valley, AZ 85253
(602) 951-8985

Founded in 1990 by a psychotherapist and two bereavement specialists to help the children who are the "neglected bereaved" when a death occurs, program provides child and adult support groups that meet twice monthly and use discussion and play activities to deal with such grief issues as anger, isolation, and guilt. Groups are facilitated by volunteers who complete a thirty-hour, eight-week training course (on child development, mental health, bereavement) taught by mental health professionals. Adults and children join in dinner, then attend separate groups that run concurrently. Program has four adult and nine children's groups. Develops educational resources for other professionals, including school counselors, social workers, bereaved family members.

California

H.O.P.E. Project (Hands Outstretched for Positive Empowerment)
c/o Legal Services for Children
1254 Market St., 3d Floor
San Francisco, CA 94102
(415) 863-3762

Provides case management services to help affected families secure supportive services in the community, emergency respite care, day care, and guardianship planning. Uses social worker-attorney teams to help parents write plans for custody. Claims to run sole support group for affected children living in families with AIDS in San Francisco.

Sunburst National AIDS Projects
P.O. Box 2824
Petaluma, CA 94953
(707) 769-0169   (707) 763-6427, fax

Runs Camp Sunburst, a weeklong residential summer camp for children infected by HIV and their families. Maintains 1:1 camper-to-counselor ratio. Free camperships (includes airfare) provided to the infected child and a parent or sibling. (Number of camperships available each year depends on donations.) First camp for HIV-affected families in country, established in 1988. Families come from all over the country. Has special director for the "sibling program" which helps meet needs of the affected siblings. One evening a week families join in "Messages from the Heart," a therapeutic arts program that has produced a moving cassette recording of songs written during this program by child and adult campers.

Florida

Tampa AIDS Network
11215 N. Nebraska Ave., Suite B-3
Tampa, FL 33612
(813) 978-8683, information   (813) 978-3515, fax

Provides weekly support groups for: (*a*) parents and children to age four; (*b*) affected children ages five to twelve (a weekly fun activity, with volunteers providing transportation and supervision); (*c*) affected youths ages thirteen to twenty-one (social activities, grief work, life skills training). Uses a "memory group" facilitator, and provides individual and family counseling. Francis House Children's Programs help meet emotional needs of affected children through creative expression (art, music, play), supervised by professional staff and volunteers. Publishes statewide, bimonthly newsletter by, for, and about women and children with HIV. Florida Women's AIDS Resource Movement (WARM) targets women of childbearing age and teens with education, support groups.

Georgia

AID Atlanta
1438 W. Peachtree St. NW, Suite 100
Atlanta, GA 30309-3624
(404) 872-0600   (404) 885-6799, fax

Runs group for affected teens, day care center for children of infected mothers, a "Buddy Junior" program, a "Care Network Program" (to help organize a client's support network of family, friends, and caregivers to ensure all needs are met), and special events for whole families (spring carnival at the zoo, for example). Asks therapists to donate time to counsel affected children and their families.

Illinois

Second Family Program
Lutheran Social Services of Illinois
6525 W. North Avenue, Suite 212
Oak Park, IL 60302-1019
(708) 445-8341   (708) 445-8351, fax

Established in 1993 to help HIV-infected parents find adoptive families or guardians for their children. Program recruits "second" families, who attend eight-week training program about the grief children experience when losing their parents and how to smooth the transition. Once the birth mother has selected a second family, program assists the two families in building a solid relationship (giving the child psychological permission from the ill parent to attach to this new family). Children are placed with families near their homes, so that child can remain with the ill parent as long as possible; the second family provides respite care in times of illness. Program also helps families locate health services, substance abuse treatment, financial assistance, and legal counsel. Social workers counsel parents concerning children's needs and run support groups. If children are placed outside immediate family, program helps ensure contact with extended family members. Adoption process is less restrictive (no adoption fees, no restrictions on marital status, income, and employment status of prospective adoptive parents, but they must qualify to be licensed foster parents, unless from child's immediate family). One hurdle: adopting parents are not currently eligible for an adoption subsidy.

New Jersey

Teen Community Center
Horizon Health Center
708 Bergen Ave.
Jersey City, NJ 07306
(201) 451-6300

For youths ages twelve to twenty-four, Center has meeting and counseling rooms, kitchen, theater/dance rehearsal rooms, craft room, pool table. Provides range of programs, including: Teen Bereavement Group (staffed by psychologist and social worker); TNT (Teens and Theatre, a semi-professional teen peer educator theater group); The Choice is Mine Group (for nonparenting teens); F.I.N.E. Group (for pregnant women under twenty); Young Mother's Group; Young Father's Group; and Food Service Training (runs own catering service). Has an Adopt-A-Teen program: teens sign pledge to stay in school, provide volunteer service, attend teen support groups at Horizon, avoid drugs/alcohol and adult sponsor pledges $25 per month for costs of teen's transportation, cultural experiences, refreshments, etc.

New York

Community Consultation Center
Henry Street Settlement
40 Montgomery St.
New York, NY 10002
(212) 233-5032

See description in Chapter 8.

Family Center for Services and Research
66 Reade St., Fifth Floor
New York, NY 10007
(212) 766-4522

See description in Chapter 8.

Special Needs Clinic at Babies Hospital
Columbia-Presbyterian Medical Center
622 W. 168th St.
New York, NY 10032

(212) 305-3093

See description in Chapter 8.

Well Children in AIDS Families Project
Beth Israel Medical Center
First Avenue and East 16th Street
New York, NY 10003
(212) 420-2851

See description in Chapter 8.

Washington

Rise n' Shine
1305 Fourth Ave.
910 Cobb Building
Seattle, WA 98101
(206) 628-8949

Started in 1988, Rise n' Shine runs programs for children living with HIV disease, children with parents, siblings, or close relatives living with HIV disease, and children orphaned by AIDS. The Love a Child program connects a trained volunteer with a child who needs emotional support. The adult provides opportunities for play and learning and gives supplemental love and attention. Its Magic Circle program runs two weekly support groups (for children aged six to nine and aged nine to thirteen), which use art, music, and dance to help children convey their feelings and which teach children about AIDS and how to deal with the death and dying around them. The Kid's Services and Special Activities program provides a range of services to children, from transportation to visit a hospitalized parent to new experiences that let the children "just be kids"—summer camp, trips, and holiday and birthday parties.

Wisconsin

The Camp Heartland Project
4565 N. Green Bay Ave.
Milwaukee, WI 53209
(414) 374-2267 or 354-5554   (414) 354-7334, fax

Founded in the summer of 1993 by a man in his early twenties and a group of student volunteers, the project provides summer camping sessions for children ages five to eighteen who are infected by HIV, their brothers and sisters, and children whose parents have died of AIDS. In 1994 several hundred children from over thirty states attended camp in rented facilities in New

Jersey, Wisconsin, and California. The three-week camp session includes a week of counselor training and ten days of camp for the children, followed by a shorter family camp when parents join their children. The camp subsidizes all of the children's transportation and camp costs through charitable donations. The project also operates a peer education program, the Camp Heartland AIDS Awareness Campaign, in which children with HIV disease address students from middle and high schools and answer questions about their experiences. As a result of these presentations, which reach three thousand students monthly, several dozen college and high school chapters of Students for Camp Heartland have developed, providing AIDS education in the schools and conducting fund-raisers to help send children to camp. The weeklong Camp Heartland Comprehensive HIV/AIDS Youth Training Program trains high school and college students to be peer AIDS educators.

Contributors

Jean Adnopoz, M.P.H.

Jean Adnopoz is associate clinical professor and coordinator of community child development and child welfare at the Child Study Center at Yale University. She has lectured and published widely on a variety of topics concerning the psychological well-being of children and the preservation of families. Her recent publications (with Steven Nagler) concerning AIDS include chapters in *Child and Adolescent Psychiatry: A Comprehensive Textbook* (Williams and Wilkins, 1990), *Advancing Family Preservation Practice* (Sage, 1992), and *Psychiatry* (Lippincott, 1992). She is a graduate of Wellesley College and the Yale School of Medicine, Department of Epidemiology and Public Health.

Gary R. Anderson, Ph.D., M.S.W.

Gary Anderson is a professor at the Hunter College School of Social Work, City University of New York. He received his Ph.D. from the University of Chicago's School of Social Service Administration. For the Child Welfare League of America, he has written *Children and AIDS: The Challenge for Child Welfare* (1986) and edited *Courage to Care: Responding to the Crisis of Children with AIDS* (1990). He has also published many other chapters and articles on the response of the child welfare system to HIV-infected children.

Warren A. Andiman, M.D.

Warren Andiman is professor of pediatrics and epidemiology at Yale University School of Medicine. Since July 1988 he has been director of the Pediatric AIDS Program at Yale-New Haven Hospital. Between July 1986 and

June 1991, he was also the first incumbent medical director of the AIDS Care Program at Yale-New Haven Hospital. Dr. Andiman has received grant support from both the American Foundation for AIDS Research (AmFAR) and the National Institutes of Health to study various aspects of the epidemiology, natural history, and virology of pediatric AIDS and has published extensively on AIDS in children. He received the Liberty Bell Award from the New Haven County Bar Association for his pioneering work, and serves on the Scientific Advisory Committee of AmFAR and the Pediatric AIDS Foundation.

Roberta J. Apfel, M.D., M.P.H.

Roberta Apfel is associate professor of clinical psychiatry at the Cambridge Hospital, Harvard Medical School, and a member of the faculty at the Boston Psychoanalytic Institute. She is codirector (with Bennett Simon, M.D.) of the Children in War Project and coeditor of a forthcoming Yale University Press book on children in war and situations of violence. Her research in Israel with Palestinian and Israeli child war survivors is ongoing. In Boston, she works with persons living with AIDS, including many women with children.

Adaline DeMarrais, M.A.

Adaline DeMarrais is a psychotherapist who first started working with children whose parents had AIDS ten years ago. She founded and directs Evergreen Network, Inc., in Southport, Connecticut, which provides support services to more than one hundred children living with HIV disease in their families. As a part of her support groups for the uninfected children, "The Sunshine Kids," she frequently asks children to express their feelings through art.

Barbara Hermie Draimin, D.S.W.

Barbara Draimin is the director of planning and community affairs for the Division of AIDS Services for the New York City Human Resources Administration, responsible for analyzing, evaluating, and planning city services for persons with AIDS. She has been principal investigator on state and federal grants funding services to AIDS-affected children and families and is an adjunct instructor in the Hunter College School of Social Work Post Masters Program in Administration. She has recently published *Coping When a Parent Has AIDS* (New York: Rosen, 1993), *The Mental Health Needs of Well Adolescents in Families with AIDS* (with J. Hudis and J. Segura, New York: New York City Human Resources Administration, 1992), and "Adolescents in Families with AIDS: Growing Up with Loss," in *A Death in the Family: Orphans of the AIDS Epidemic,* ed. Carol Levine (New York: United Hospital Fund, 1993).

Brian W. C. Forsyth, M.B., Ch.B., F.R.C.P.(C.)

Brian Forsyth is associate professor of pediatrics at the Child Study Center at Yale University, an attending pediatrician in the Pediatric AIDS Program at Yale-New Haven Hospital, and medical director of the Family Support Program for HIV-Affected Children at the Child Study Center. He is a graduate of Glasgow University and completed his pediatric residency at Montreal Children's Hospital. Dr. Forsyth is an active participant in developing services in the community for persons with AIDS and works with others in developing policies to address the needs of those affected by AIDS.

Shelley Diehl Geballe, J.D.

Shelley Geballe is a civil rights attorney, currently in the doctoral program in health policy in the Department of Epidemiology and Public Health at Yale University School of Medicine. While associate legal director for the ACLU in Connecticut, she brought successful class action litigation challenging the exclusion of children with HIV disease from the New Haven Public Schools, inadequate health care for Connecticut inmates with HIV disease, and systemic deficiencies in Connecticut's child welfare system. A graduate of Yale Law School, she taught "AIDS and the Law" with Harlon Dalton while on its faculty and is currently a professor of law (adjunct) at the University of Connecticut Law School. She lectures frequently on AIDS-related legal issues.

Nora Ellen Groce, Ph.D.

Nora Groce is an assistant professor in the Department of Epidemiology and Public Health at Yale Medical School. A medical anthropologist, she was founder and director of the Cross-Cultural Program at the Newington Children's Hospital. Her work has focused on issues of ethnic and minority children's health within the American medical system, as well as on issues of disability and chronic disease viewed cross-culturally. She is the author of three books and a number of journal articles, including "Culture and Chronic Illness: Raising Children with Disabling Conditions in a Culturally Diverse World," published in *Pediatrics* in 1993.

Janice M. Gruendel, Ph.D.

Janice Gruendel is currently vice president of Rabbit Ears Productions, a children's multimedia publishing company in Connecticut, and head of the Education Group. With Connecticut Public Television, she is co–executive producer of *Mommy, Who'll Take Care of Me?*, a videodocumentary on children living with AIDS in their families. Before joining Rabbit Ears, she served the State of Connecticut for thirteen years in such positions as deputy commissioner within the Departments of Children and Youth Services, Health

Services, and Mental Retardation, and as director of health services within the Department of Corrections. She has published in both the popular and academic press and has lectured frequently on the need for systems reform in order to better meet the needs of children and families.

Jan Hudis, M.P.H.

Jan Hudis is program development director for The Family Center in New York City, which provides services to terminally ill parents, their children, and their new guardians. She is involved in design and implementation of a federally funded four-year intervention study of adolescents in families with AIDS. With Barbara Draimin, she wrote *The Mental Health Needs of Well Adolescents in Families with AIDS* (New York: New York City Human Resources Division, 1992), the final report of a study funded by the National Institute of Mental Health.

Carol Levine, M.A.

Carol Levine is executive director of The Orphan Project: Families and Children in the HIV Epidemic, administered by the Fund for the City of New York. She was formerly executive director of the Citizens Commission on AIDS, a foundation-supported group dedicated to stimulating leadership on AIDS in New York City and Northern New Jersey. Before joining the commission in 1987, she was on the staff of the Hastings Center, a nonprofit research and education institute in the field of medical ethics. She is editor of *Taking Sides: Controversial Issues in Biomedical Ethics* (5th ed., Guilford, Conn.: Dushkin, 1993), and *A Death in the Family: Orphans of the HIV Epidemic* (New York: United Hospital Fund, 1993). She is coeditor with Barbara Dane of *AIDS and the New Orphans: Coping with Death* (Greenwood, 1994). Ms. Levine was awarded a MacArthur Fellowship in 1993.

Melvin Lewis, M.B.B.S., F.R.C.Psych, D.U.H.

Melvin Lewis is professor of pediatrics and psychiatry at the Child Study Center at Yale University, attending in pediatrics and child psychiatry at Yale-New Haven Hospital, and principal investigator for the Uninfected Children of HIV Affected Families program at the Yale Child Study Center and Yale-New Haven Hospital. He is a graduate of Guy's Hospital Medical School, London University, and completed his residencies in pediatrics, psychiatry, and child psychiatry at Yale. Dr. Lewis is also a child psychoanalyst, and is the editor of *Child and Adolescent Psychiatry: A Comprehensive Textbook.*

Steven F. Nagler, M.S.W., A.C.S.W.

Steven Nagler is clinical director of the Family Support Service and Assistant Clinical Professor in Social Work at the Child Study Center at Yale University. He has developed programs with Ms. Adnopoz and written extensively about home- and community-based programs that provide mental health and casework services to vulnerable children and their families. He also maintains a private practice of adult and child psychotherapy. He is a graduate of Amherst College and the Smith College School for Social Work.

Alvin Novick, M.D.

Alvin Novick is professor of biology at Yale University and an ethicist dealing especially with HIV-related issues. Since 1982, Dr. Novick has devoted full-time effort to the social and political aspects of AIDS, including developing prevention, care, and residence programs for gay men, injection drug users, sex workers, the minority poor, women, and children. He chaired the drive in Connecticut for New Haven's needle exchange program and for a national program to counsel and rehabilitate HIV-infected health care providers. He is currently editor-in-chief of the *AIDS and Public Policy Journal* and the cochairperson of a national planning committee seeking to develop and implement a second wave of enlightened HIV prevention efforts, drawing on a decade of experience with AIDS prevention.

June E. Osborn, M.D.

June Osborn is professor of epidemiology in the School of Public Health and Professor of Pediatrics and Communicable Diseases in the School of Medicine at the University of Michigan. Between 1984 and 1993, she served as dean of Michigan's School of Public Health, and between 1989 and 1993 she was the chairman of the United States National Commission on AIDS. In the past eight years, she has published more than forty articles on AIDS and its impact and has been a consultant on AIDS-related issues to many organizations, including WHO's Global Commission on AIDS (1988–92) and the Steering Committee of the Global AIDS Policy Coalition (Jonathan Mann, chairman).

Cynthia J. Telingator, M.D.

Cynthia Telingator is an instructor in psychiatry at the Cambridge Hospital, Harvard Medical School. She completed her training in adult and child psychiatry at the Cambridge Hospital. A child, adolescent, and adult psychiatrist, she has a private practice and is developing a program at the Zinberg HIV Clinic at Cambridge Hospital to focus on the needs of children and families affected by HIV disease. She has presented her clinical work with families affected by HIV at the annual meeting of the American Academy of Child and Adolescent Psychiatrists.

Index